wx 173   20.46

Implementing an El Medical Record Sys

successes, failures, lessons

Tim Scott
Senior Lecturer in Organisation
School of Management
University of St Andrews, Fife

Thomas G Rundall
Henry J. Kaiser Professor of Organized Health Systems
School of Public Health
University of California, Berkeley

Thomas M Vogt
Program Director
Kaiser Permanente Center for Health Research
Hawaii

John Hsu
Physician Scientist
Kaiser Permanente Division of Research
Oakland, California

Foreword by

Jos Aarts

Radcliffe Publishing
Oxford • Seattle

Radcliffe Publishing Ltd
18 Marcham Road
Abingdon
Oxon OX14 1AA
United Kingdom

www.radcliffe-oxford.com
Electronic catalogue and worldwide online ordering facility.

British Library Cataloguing in Publication Data

A catalogue record for this book is available from the British Library.

ISBN-10   1 85775 750 5
ISBN-13   978 1 85775 750 7

Typeset by Ann Buchan (Typesetters), Middlesex, UK
Printed and bound by Biddles Ltd, King's Lynn, Norfolk, UK

Contents

Foreword   vii
Preface   ix
Acknowledgements   xi

1 **Introduction**   1
The international context   1
Research context   2
Potential benefits of EMR and evidence   3
EMRs and chronic disease management   5
Hawaii Kaiser Permanente   6
A History of Kaiser Permanente   7
   Mojave Desert: 1933–1938   8
   Grand Coulee: 1938–1941   10
   World War II and the shipyards: 1942–1945   11
   Survival and reorganisation in the post-war era: 1946–1951 14
   The struggle for control: 1952–1955   17
   The Tahoe Agreement: 1955–1960   21
   Regional Management Teams   23
   Kaiser Permanente in Hawaii   25
   1960s–present: a model for American healthcare?   28
Methodology   30
   Qualitative research   30
   Validity and reliability   32
   Method   34

2 **The experience of implementation**   35
Introduction   35
   Summary of implementation   36
The implementation process: CIS development   36
   Delayed implementation start date   36
   Product design issues   37
   CIS development: getting changes made in the CIS software 39
Care delivery issues: nothing and everything to do with CIS   43
   Identity and access   44
   Scope of practice   45
Loss of flexibility   47
The electronic In-Basket   49
   Heterogeneous responses to the In-Basket   49

Templates   51
Care process innovation   54
E-conversion   54
MD telephone triage   55
Automation, integration or transformation?   56
CIS in context: one among many tools   58
Other benefits of CIS implementation   59
    The Electronic Medical Record   59
    Accountability   60
    Decision making   62
    Interagency communication   63
    Quality   64
    The visit is not the visit   65
    Chronic disease management   67
    Other lessons learned from implementing CIS   68
Summary of reported experience of CIS   69

3 Accounting for successes and failures   **71**
The decision to adopt CIS   71
CIS in Colorado and Hawaii   72
Who was to blame?   73
Organisational culture   75
    Clinic cultures   77
    Specialty subcultures   78
    Cultures and implementation   80
Leadership   82
The approach to implementation   89
Was the first site a pilot?   92
Workflow analysis   93
Readiness   96
    Specialty differences   96
    E-literacy   98
    Size   98
Healthcare teams   99
User responses to CIS   101
    Training and support   101
    Aptitude   103
Implementation team management   104
Time burden   106
The impact of previous IT innovation   109
Resistance   111
Conflict   112
    Personal conflict   112
    Regional–national conflict   113
    Conflict between Kaiser Permanente and IBM   115
    Conflict between medical and nursing staff   116
Conclusion   116

4   Barriers and facilitators to implementation   118
   Summary of findings   118
      Failures   119
      Successes   119
   The adoption decision   120
   Technical problems   121
   Approaches to implementation   122
   Training and support   123
   Specialty differences   123
   A great magnifier   124
   CIS team management   124
   Nothing and everything to do with CIS   125
   The time burden   125
   Healthcare teams   126
   Organisational culture   126
   Leadership   128
   Resistance   130
   Impact of previous information and communication technology
   implementations   131
   Conflict   131
   Success, failure or learning experience?   132
   Wider implications   133

5   Electronic medical record systems: lessons for   134
   implementation
   State of EMR implementation   134
   Key processes   135
      Choosing the right EMR for adoption   135
      Dealing with initial software design problems   135
      Managing impact on clinician productivity   136
      Managing changing clinical roles and responsibilities   136
      Managing frustrations, resistance and conflict   137
      Anticipating culturally informed responses   137
      Promoting responsive leadership   137
      Implementation models   138
      Complex adaptive model   139
      Catching a wave   139
   Limitations of the study   140
      Validity of interview data   140
      Success and failure revisited   141

Appendix A: Facilitators and barriers to IT implementation   142
and its effects on clinical care design

References   148
Index   153

Foreword

Books about the implementation of information systems in health care organizations are rare. Tim Scott and his colleagues have written such a rare book. It is easy to write a report about the failure of a technology and identify culprits. In terms of such a report the implementation of the information system that the author describes is a failure. It never got to work in the medical work practices that it was supposed to support. But Dr. Scott and his co-authors refrain from identifying culprits. They even posit that the failed implementation was a success because it prepared the organization for how to deal with the introduction of new technologies that are so pervasive. In their view essential to the success of an implementation is the degree of organizational learning that occurs.

Dr. Scott and his colleagues carefully researched and documented the history of the implementation of an electronic medical record system in a US health maintenance organization. They have spent enough time to become sensitive to its specific organizational and cultural context and yet remained careful observers enabling them to describe and analyze their findings.

Their observations and findings are important for both researchers and practitioners. They do not offer a cookbook on how to implement a clinical information system successfully. Rather they let the facts speak for themselves and leave room for the reader to make her own conclusions. Yet, the authors present interesting conclusions and challenge accepted wisdom. For example, IT makes the invisible visible and they show how the introduction of the electronic medical record made visible the informally accepted scope of practice of nurses and medical assistants and how formal procedures had to be established to align the scope with legal regulations and still make medical work doable. They show that "one size fits all" does not work, because different medical specialties have different ways of dealing with patients and that across the organization even the same medical specialties deal differently with patients depending on their backgrounds and local customs. No one questions the need for proper training when introducing IT, but Dr. Scott and colleagues raise the question whether training should be focused on how to use a system or how to practise medicine better with the new IT tools. This observation highlights a very important aspect of this book: the awareness that the implementation of clinical IT should not just support existing practices but should play a crucial role in the discussion of how to make medical practice better. The fact that the increased workload of using the electronic medical record redefined the necessity of seeing all patients in the office is a case in point. The authors challenge the accepted wisdom that emphasizes the need for organizational leadership to implement IT. They argue that leadership could very well emerge from a largely unconscious response to events, which in hindsight could be labeled as such. Their carefully documented case shows how many events unfolded unexpectedly and required the actors to improvise their responses in a way that Claudio Ciborra calls 'bricolage'*, a response that helped them to appropriate a system and is still innovative. I think Dr. Scott and his co-authors are right when they doubt whether a checklist of technical and organizational variables is useful to assess how IT as an innovation will affect an organization.

I recommend this book to everyone who wants to make a serious study of the implementation of IT in complex organizations, not only in the healthcare field but also in the wider community of information systems.

Dr. Jos Aarts
Senior Research Scientist
Erasmus University Rotterdam
September 2006

---

*Ciborra C (2002) The labyrinths of information, challenging the wisdom of systems. Oxford, Oxford University Press

Preface

Ethnography is bound up with travelling, both literally and metaphorically. Travelling to foreign lands has always been both an adventure and a metaphor for adventure – no one can predict what will befall the traveller – it is an inherently unpredictable activity. Few, perhaps, are lucky enough to combine research and travel in such pleasant lands as northern California and Hawaii. But the reader should not be fooled by the exoticness of the setting, nor the workday character of the intervention studied. The wider applicability of the lessons related here is inherently and insolubly problematic, research findings are rarely automatically transferable to different settings. But the successes, failures and lessons do contain important information for health systems planning to introduce new information technology to improve healthcare.

There is, after all, a constant urge to illuminate one's own experience in the light of the experiences of others. This is doubtless one reason why biographies and autobiographies are fascinating. We gain a certain distance between self as observer and self as subject. There is a constant tension between the will to go forth and discover what is strange and unfamiliar for its own sake, and for what it can reveal about ourselves and our culture – which for many of us is so familiar as to seem not to exist. In this double process we begin to see the other in our terms and hopefully ourselves in the others' terms. But whether we can ever see ourselves in our own terms, or the other in the other's terms is yet to be demonstrated as far as we are aware.

Innovation is like travelling in negative. Instead of the familiar entering the foreign system, innovation is the foreign entering the familiar system, like receiving a stranger in one's midst, or a virus into one's body – the traveller as other. The stranger is another constant in literature as in our life world. How does one deal with the stranger, who is always abnormal and disturbing? One begins to see how impossibly complex innovation research can be: an investigator proceeds to study the foreign inserted into the familiar setting, but a familiar setting not necessarily his own. In other words: a foreigner studying a foreign intervention into a foreign familiar. Then one recalls that every study is an intervention in itself. Paradox piled upon paradox.

One can only begin, therefore, at the beginning. One can only write narrative. We heard that a certain process had occurred. We went to see for ourselves, and ask the local people what they had seen. We made some notes and came home to write an account. That is all.

In this case the notes made were recordings of conversations. To the ethnographer a conversation is more than a data collection exercise – it is a beautiful event; an inexhaustible signifier which no writing can truly measure up to or account for. One recalls all such conversations with a poignant mixture of pleasure and regret. One usually sees the best of people in these hours: thoughtful, candid, sympathetic, reflective, articulate, passionate. The research interview is often and for both individuals a time-out from the urgent, oppressive and con-flicting demands of their workaday lives. It is even sometimes therapeutic; an unintended consequence of the conscious mind reviewing events and restoring them in a slightly better order. This is the fundamental human faculty of organi-sation at work. This account draws on such conversations liberally, reproducing many excerpts. So far as possible, therefore, this book is an account of how Hawaii Kaiser Permanente tried to implement a clinical information system in the par-ticipants' own words. As a piece of ethnography it is inevitably partial and may contain biases that we are not aware of. Whatever they are, they are ultimately ours and no one else's.

In Hawaii, the birthplace of surfing, there is a certain phrase – 'Catching a wave' – innovations like electronic information and communication technolo-gies occur in waves not dissimilar to the constant swells running across the surface layers of the Pacific Ocean, rearing up as waves on reaching Hawaii's reefs, and breaking onto its many beaches. The career of CIS in Hawaii is the wave, Hawaii Kaiser Permanente the reef, and the doctors, nurses, administra-tors and others surfers immersed in the swell off their particular local beaches, waiting to catch the wave. 'It was,' as one respondent commented wryly, 'a wild ride'.

Tim Scott
Thomas G Rundall
John Hsu
September 2006

Acknowledgements

This research was conceived, designed and conducted whilst Tim Scott was a Harkness Fellow in Health Policy, funded by The Commonwealth Fund of New York, and a Visiting Scholar at the University of California, Berkeley, 2002–3, for which thanks to the School of Public Health at Berkeley. The Garfield Foundation provided funding for the data collection. The original report on which this book is based was completed at the University of York, thanks to Trevor Sheldon's patience and support. James Kinsman at Kaiser Permanente Division of Research, Oakland, California contributed to the administration of the study. Geoffrey Galbraith and Kathy Mau, at Hawaii Kaiser Permanente, contributed to the recruitment of participants and administration of the study. Judy Li, at the University of California, Berkeley, and SRI International, validated the interview transcripts. We thank all those Kaiser Permanente employees who participated so frankly and generously in our study.

Finally, to Lesline, Kanani, Kathryn, Max, Noe and Brent in Waimanalo, Oahu, who showed us the wider meaning of catching a wave: *Mahalo Nui Loa!*

Chapter 1

Introduction

The international context

Healthcare delivery systems in some countries such, as the USA, UK, Sweden and Hong Kong, have made limited progress with the use of electronic medical records (EMRs). EMRs are also being developed for the Canadian and Australian health systems. However, none of the existing or planned EMRs has the scale envisaged for the EMR currently being implemented by the UK National Health Service.[17,30,59] The NHS National Programme for Information Technology (NPfIT), is currently budgeted at over £6 billion and projected to cost in excess of £20 billion over the next 10 years. It is therefore one of the most expensive civilian programs of any kind to be mounted anywhere. It features a national electronic medical record and integrated functions including documentation, care management, ordering, messaging, analysis and reporting, access to knowledge resources and patient website access. Whilst national and local service provider contracts have been awarded, the task of implementation is still nascent. The risk of failure remains high due to the undeveloped state of the technology and the organisational challenges involved in implementation. The NHS 'has had its share of failed health information systems, wasted millions and disciplinary hearings'.[4,47,55] Other large, integrated healthcare organisations, like Kaiser Permanente, may provide useful insights to help the NHS achieve higher levels of adoption, acceptance and use.

Despite frequent calls in the US for greater use of EMRs,[33,34,36] adoption of such technology has been limited.[53,54] Few large systems have introduced or evaluated an EMR, partly due to the difficulty of the task and the lack of clear 'best practices' for implementation. Most of what is known about the implementation of EMRs comes from five benchmark institutions: the Regenstrief Institute; Brigham and Women's Hospital/Partners Health Care; the Department of Veterans Affairs; LDS Hospital/Intermountain Health Care; and Kaiser Permanente. Based on the experience of these institutions, it is clear that adopting new IT is a major challenge in healthcare organisations.[15] Success appears to be determined more by organisational than technical factors, though research to date is just beginning to identify specific organisational factors that facilitate or impede EMR implementation.[1,41,61] Another reason for the slow uptake is a lack of convincing evidence that EMR adoption improves either the quality or efficiency of care. Though some studies have found positive evidence of the benefits of EMRs on care processes and health and financial outcomes,[17] others have found disappointingly small or no effects on quality or costs.[24,39,47] Healthcare systems already facing significant financial constraints have tended to avoid the high costs and uncertain returns of implementing an EMR.[20,21] And such projects face complex organisational challenges to integrate the new technology into workflows and redesign care processes to harness its potential.[11,54]

Research context

There are seven main reasons why a new, IT-based medical care paradigm is emerging:

1 A paper-based system to support clinical care is increasingly non-viable.
2 Human memory-based medicine is increasingly unreliable.
3 Clinical data capture has become a business imperative.
4 Consumer expectations for improved care and service are rising.[61]
5 The prevalence of chronic diseases is steadily rising, requiring closer monitoring of patients and greater coordination of care.
6 Public and private sector payers are demanding more accountability from providers for the cost of care, quality of care, and patient outcomes.
7 New technologies make it possible to evaluate and intervene to improve care in ways not heretofore possible.

These points encapsulate a number of important trends witnessed over the past 50 years. Evidence-based medicine (EBM) is supplanting traditional and parochial clinical training and practice. Diagnostic and treatment decisions are increasingly based on the results of clinical trials interpreted in a community medicine context. A parallel development is the increasing demand for epidemiologists to apply statistical methods to study health and illness at the population level to guide healthcare and other agencies. To help to disseminate the exponential growth in medical knowledge, many professional biomedical journals are now published on the Internet, improving accessibility for computer-literate clinicians and consumers. But it has become virtually impossible for clinicians to read and retain all the knowledge available even in their own fields. A new approach to processing information is therefore needed to facilitate access to relevant information for effective and efficient care management at the point of care. Such systems need to help clinicians discriminate between 'signal' and 'noise'. As multiple specialties may be involved in caring for individual patients, it is also likely that the clinical team rather than the individual clinician will be involved in information processing, decision making and other aspects of care management.

Though IT innovations have the potential to improve healthcare quality, integration and efficiency,[7,33,34] they require large capital investments in an industry with significant financial constraints. A clearer understanding of the value of these innovations is essential to inform diffusion of information technology in the current healthcare environment. Understanding how providers actually use each functional component of the systems and which components create value are crucial issues not adequately answered by the literature.[31,34] This type of information may also be crucial to improvements in other critical areas such as patient safety and overall care for vulnerable populations, including patients with chronic disease or members of underserved ethnic groups.

In 1991 the Institute of Medicine (IOM) recognised the potential of a computer-based record to support evidence-based care, quality improvement and evaluation; and called for the computer-based patient record to become a standard health technology by 2001.[33] Since 1991 further reports have described serious concerns about healthcare delivery, including a high incidence of preventable errors, disparities in care delivery between different ethnic groups, and a need to redesign systems and infrastructure to achieve quality improvements.[5,9,19,21,41,67] In *Crossing the Quality Chasm*, the IOM specifically targeted information technology as a key agent for change, an enabling structural innovation:

> *The committee believes IT must play a central role in the redesign of the healthcare system if substantial improvement in healthcare quality is to be achieved during the coming decade...the importance of a strong information infrastructure in supporting efforts to reengineer care processes...coordinate patient care across clinicians and settings and overtime, support multidisciplinary team functioning, and facilitate performance and outcome measurement for improvement and accountability.*[34]

Designing and implementing an electronic medical record presents social as well as technical and financial challenges. It has been estimated, albeit loosely, that the IT innovation challenge is 20% technological and 80% sociological. Implied changes are far-reaching in terms of revised roles, status, responsibilities and relationships, which all need to be seen as part of a qualitative shift from a closed system model of healthcare, where decisions are traditionally informed by the individual expertise of clinicians, to a more open model, where decision making is informed by a number of sources both inside and outside the consulting room. These are likely to include a clinical team as opposed to a sole provider, the patient and significant others, the health record, alerts, evidence of trials and meta-analyses, and data accessed via the Internet. A well-designed EMR could be the hub of this information, supporting safer, more effective and efficient care management, but only if clinicians are ready and able to integrate it into different models of care and clinical practice. One aim of this book is to reflect on cultural influences on the implementation of an EMR in Hawaii Kaiser Permanente.

Potential benefits of EMR and evidence

Electronic medical record or EMR is a generic term for integrated, computer-based, health information systems, accessible at the point of care. A typical EMR will be multifunctional, including an electronic patient health record updated in real time by information inputted at any workstation or other interface connected to a secure network. An EMR also has information management tools to provide clinical reminders and alerts, review lab results, link with knowledge sources for healthcare decision making, and analysis of aggregate data. An EMR extends the usefulness of patient data by the application of information management tools.[78] Typical electronic medical records include some or all of the components in Table 1.1.

The potential benefits of EMRs correspond to the type and number of functions they can perform. However, there have been relatively few studies of the benefits of IT innovations in healthcare of *any* kind. Most of the tangible evidence on IT relates to computer decision support systems (CDSS). Hunt *et al.*

Table 1.1. Components of electronic medical records

Function/Application	Description
Practitioner order entry: • laboratory management • pharmacy management • diagnostic imaging management • referral management • decision support • alerts	To support ordering laboratory tests, drug prescribing, diagnostic imaging or consult requests. Decision support and alerts are typically integrated into order entry capabilities.
Electronic patient record	Integrated storage and presentation of patient information.
Document management	To allow clinicians to record, in code or text, the actions they have taken in diagnosing, managing and treating a patient. This could include physician and nursing progress notes and the medication administration record.
Clinical decision support	Alerts based on current data from the electronic medical record, evidence-based practice guidelines, or more complex artificial intelligence systems for diagnostic support provided at the time the clinician is formulating an assessment of the patient's condition and making ordering decisions.
Administrative data	Access to administrative data such as admission, discharge and transfer records, surgery schedules, demographic data, room assignments, etc.
Integrated communication support	Tools that facilitate effective and efficient communication among team members (including the patient) to support continuity of care among multiple providers.
Access to knowledge resources	Online information, including reference materials, journal articles, guidelines, etc., at the time decisions are being made regarding patient care.

Adapted from Raymond and Dold.[61]

reviewed 68 controlled trials of CDSS and found that drug dosing support and preventative care support both appear to have demonstrable benefits, whereas there is little evidence for diagnostic decision support.[31] The review found a dearth of studies that measured effects on patient outcomes, and instead focused on intermediate factors such as potential medication errors. Most studies were of inpatient settings and did not include outpatient care.

Bates *et al.* assessed the introduction of a computer order entry system for inpatient medication to improve communication between physicians, pharmacists, and nurses.[8] The intervention permitted closer integration of clinical services between providers, and simplified the clinical processes, e.g. elimination of a medication order transcriber. The study also found a significant decrease in serious medication errors (55%), and a decrease in transcription errors (84%). In a similar study, Evans *et al.* evaluated a computerised antibiotic management program.[20] At post-test, significant decreases in potential errors were found, e.g. allergic contraindications, excess dosages, excessive drug exposure time, adverse events associated with medications, and higher quality of care, e.g. better antibiotic-susceptibility matching. In a study of a computer reminder system, Demarkis *et al.* assessed the use of IT to increase the coherence and uniformity of care across multiple primary care providers.[16] The study found that computer reminders increased adherence with clinical recommendations, but that the adherence rate decreased to the baseline rate within one year.

Robinson reviewed the state of communication studies and described the findings of the Science Panel on Interactive Communication and Health (SciPICH), convened by the Office of Disease Prevention and Health Promotion of the US Department of Health and Human Services.[62] The panel concluded that although interactive health communication has great potential to improve patient learning and health communication, there are also significant potential harms associated with misinformation. However, the panel found few studies that had rigorously evaluated patient communication applications.

In addition to improving the quality of healthcare, IT has significant potential to measure performance. Tracking performance is essential to support continuous quality improvement, and permits more sophisticated purchasing and managerial decisions. However, there is a dearth of empirical data in this area. Measures of physician productivity are crude, e.g. numbers of patients seen per hour, and there have been few studies of the productivity of nursing, pharmacy or ancillary staff. There is also a dearth of studies of the timeliness of care, or the impact of EMRs on decreasing time lapse to diagnosis or effective treatment.

EMRs and chronic disease management

Two recent IOM reports identify the burden of chronic disease on patients and health systems as a US national priority for action.[35,36] Approximately 45% of people living in the United States have some type of chronic illness,[60] including asthma, diabetes, hypertension and ischaemic heart disease, stroke, depression and other severe mental illnesses.[35] Specifically, four chronic conditions affect nearly half of Americans. Asthma, depression and diabetes each affect about 15 million,[12,56,58] while five million have congestive heart failure.[38] In 1999 these four chronic diseases were directly responsible for 140 000 deaths in the United States,[29] and generated at least $173 billion in medical and other costs.[38,57,75,82] Although the effectiveness of care for patients with these and other major chronic illnesses has been improved by the use of guidelines, disease management techniques, case management and patient education,[81] many patients are not benefiting from these advances. Recent studies indicate that fewer than half of US patients with asthma, depression and diabetes receive appropriate treatment.[14,45,84] Organisational characteristics of physician practices associated with effective chronic disease care include the use of patient care teams, supportive information systems and a high volume of patients.[34]

In a US national survey of physician organisations and the management of chronic illness, Rundall *et al.* assessed the extent to which chronic care management processes (CMP) and EMRs were used to care for patients with asthma, congestive heart failure, depression and diabetes in nine large, multidisciplinary practices with national reputations for delivering high quality care (number of physicians = 147 to 2449).[65] The study also identified barriers and facilitators in these organisations that affected their ability to implement CMPs and EMRs. The care management processes studied included practice guidelines, population disease management, case management and health promotion. Information was collected on each medical group's use of seven selected functions of an EMR that support chronic disease care management: electronic patient record, recording of health history, recording of tests and procedures, recording of diagnosis and treatment, computerised entry of drug prescriptions, automated reminders and electronic exchange of information with patients. The study found that:

- 50% of physician organisations used 4 or fewer out of a possible 16 CMPs
- external incentives and information technology were the most strongly associated predictors of CMP use
- 33% of physician organisations reported no external incentives, and 50% no clinical IT capability
- external incentives and EMR technology have the potential to increase CMP use and, thereby, quality of care
- institutional facilitators and barriers to improving quality of chronic care management exist.

The study also found that use of EMR functions varied greatly among the medical groups and no group used all seven functions. The eight groups with some EMR capability used between four and six of the functions. In addition, the study found a wide variation in awareness/implementation of CMPs across chronic diseases, especially in depression. Wide variation was also found in IT capability, with only two out of fourteen sites having high levels of IT capability, of which only one (Kaiser Permanente) regarded the use of two or more CMPs as normal practice. IT capability was found to be one of the key facilitators and barriers to CMP implementation, along with good leadership, a culture valuing quality, physician champions of CMP and capitation (financial risk to provider). The relative importance of facilitators and barriers remains unclear. Hence, there is a need to examine the influence of facilitators and barriers to IT implementation and their effects on clinical care redesign in more detail.

Hawaii Kaiser Permanente

Hawaii Kaiser Permanente is one of eight regions served by Kaiser Permanente – the largest not-for-profit, integrated healthcare delivery system in the United States. Headquartered in Oakland, California, Kaiser Permanente serves over 8 million members across the US. The same general organisational model is used in each region. Doctors join regional exclusive partnerships or professional corporations that contract with the Kaiser Foundation Health Plan and assume full responsibility for providing and arranging necessary medical care for members.

Kaiser Permanente's integrated system provides all healthcare needs for adults and children, including preventative, routine, specialty, emergency, and inpatient care, ancillary testing, pharmacy, rehabilitative services, and home care.

Hawaii Kaiser Permanente has 26 primary healthcare teams in 15 clinics, and one hospital. The health system serves 234 000 members across the three largest islands in the state. The primary care teams include physicians trained in internal medicine and family practice. The healthcare providers are salaried employees of the physician professional corporation; members primarily have prepaid health benefits, i.e. fully capitated care. Nine Kaiser Permanente clinics and a hospital are located on the island of Oahu.

Since the late 1990s Kaiser Permanente has sought to create a system-wide EMR. Prior to EMR implementation in Hawaii, the health system had implemented two other comprehensive EMR systems in other regions. One system was based on a vendor-created, commercially available system. The other EMR was jointly developed between Kaiser Permanente and IBM. Hawaii's EMR was the second-generation version of the jointly developed system. The commercially produced EMR system was adopted five years earlier by Kaiser Permanente in the Northwest region (Oregon and Washington states), where it worked well. The health system experienced a change in its senior leadership. The new chief executive officer (CEO) was previously CEO of another US health system, which recently had successfully implemented the same clinical information system used by Kaiser Permanente in the Northwest.

EMR implementation was halted in Hawaii because of delays in delivering promised capacities and other problems. Hawaii Kaiser Permanente's EMR project provides an opportunity to examine the process of EMR implementation in one region of a large system and to analyse organisational factors relevant to EMR implementation.[1,23,46,48,49,77]

A History of Kaiser Permanente

In this section we present a brief history of the Kaiser Permanente medical care program, including the establishment of its Hawaii region. We have relied mainly on John G Smillie's authoritative history of the Permanente Medical Group.[72] Smillie was a Permanente physician who eventually became physician-in-chief, then assistant to the executive director.

The rise and fall of the Clinical Information System (CIS) in the Hawaii region needs to be seen in context of the Kaiser Permanente medical care program. That national program in turn has to be set in context of the history of American medicine.[76] In briefest terms, there is no comprehensive national health service in the USA. Most working Americans and their dependants are insured against ill health as an employment benefit. Others may insure their health privately with insurance companies or health plans, or even pay healthcare providers directly for their services. Persons aged 65 and older are covered by the federal Medicare health insurance program, and very low income individuals and families are eligible for health insurance benefits under Medicaid, a joint federal-state funded program. A patchwork of many other specialty health insurance programs, funded at the federal, state, and local levels – especially for children – has emerged over the past 50 years, but still many Americans fall through the cracks of these programs. It has been estimated that about 45 million people in the USA were uninsured and 16 million people aged 19–64 underinsured in 2003 (35% or 61 million in total).[66] While it is possible for an uninsured person to receive care from a private clinic or hospital as a charity patient, most uninsured people receive their medical care from county or city funded public hospitals and clinics.

It is well known that underinsured adults are more likely to delay or forgo needed care than those with adequate coverage. Obtaining healthcare in America is a serious business, not only because it has a strongly commercial character, but also because the 'system' is so fragmented. The process of registering with a physician or physicians, obtaining specific treatments from variable formularies, claiming for healthcare costs or paying for tests and treatments, can all be very complicated, frustrating and ruinously expensive. Moreover, in such a fragmented, largely private, fee-based medical care system, built upon the model of the independent physician working in solo practice, the creation of Kaiser Permanente, a new model of integrated medical care based upon prepaid group practice, was strongly opposed by traditional medical, hospital, and insurance interests. In this sense, from its very origins Kaiser Permanente has been an innovative medical institution, willing to adopt new structures, processes and technology in order to establish its niche in the American healthcare marketplace and promote its reputation as a high quality healthcare system. Kaiser Permanente's involvement with health information technology over the past several decades should be apprehended in this context.

The history of the Kaiser Permanente medical care program is surrounded by water. It was founded and developed at the construction sites of dams, aqueducts and ships; it was intimately involved in the stupendous economic development of California before, during and after World War II into an economy today estimated to be between the fifth and seventh largest in the world. It was through major construction projects to pipe water to the city of Los Angeles, the operation of ports along the US western seaboard, the Allies' dire need for ships during World War II, and the rapid postwar economic expansion of industrial communities and their healthcare needs that Kaiser Permanente emerged to become the largest privately owned health system in the USA. This history has been deeply influenced by two individuals: Sidney Garfield, MD and Henry J Kaiser.

Mojave Desert: 1933–1938

In 1933 Sidney Garfield completed his training in general surgery at Los Angeles County Hospital. He was 27 and intended to establish himself in a typical fee-for-service practice in Los Angeles. But 1933 was the worst year of the Depression and such opportunities were scarce. The ethos of medical practice in Los Angeles in which Garfield and his colleagues were educated characterised the American response to the Depression years. 'Under assault of economic hardship, the social dimension of American experience was asserting itself against an already established philosophy of individualism. These doctors were learning not only from each other and from the team at the Los Angeles County, but also from the philosophy of social responsibility that animated a great public hospital at a time of great economic stress.'[72] Garfield and his peers recognised the exceptional character of the times and fully expected to enter solo fee-for-service practice careers when the economy recovered. But their experience of group based practice at LA County helped to set a different course.

Unable to open a solo surgical practice, Garfield sought a salaried post. He learned from another Los Angeles County graduate, Gene Morris, that the Metropolitan Water District of Los Angeles was looking for a physician to staff a small medical unit at Indio on the edge of the Mojave Desert, 140 miles east of Los Angeles. The Water District was building an aqueduct from the Colorado River to Los Angeles. Garfield was offered the job but declined as he felt the $125 a month salary to be too low. Garfield and Morris decided instead to build their own small hospital at Desert Center, 60 miles east of Indio. There they would offer fee-for-service industrial medical care for on-the-job injuries and illnesses. They would also offer fee-for-service non-industrial medicine to individuals. Contractors and insurance companies said they would support the project.

Assuming an overall debt of $50 000 to get Contractors General Hospital into operation, Garfield and Morris banked on treating a high volume of insured, on-the-job injuries. They were not short of patients, who presented the full range of conditions, from fractures and infections to heart attacks and snake bites. High numbers of patients with off-the-job health problems also presented themselves, including prostitutes and their clients with syphilis and gonorrhoea. Venereal disease was considered a non-industrial illness and not covered by insurance. Earning 50 cents an hour, few individuals could pay for treatment. As there was no county hospital Garfield felt obliged to admit them, hoping that his income from indemnified injuries would tide him over. The insurance companies, however, disputed and discounted his fees, claiming overtreatment. Within seven months of opening, Contractors General Hospital faced bankruptcy.

Fortunately, the prospect of losing the CGH concentrated the minds of the contractors and insurers. The largest insurance company involved in the construction project was San Francisco-based Industrial Indemnity Exchange, established in 1921 by a group of contractors including Henry J Kaiser. Harold Hatch, chief strategist for IIE, proposed a novel method of financing medical care at CGH, by prepayment. He offered to pay 12.5% of the workers compensation insurance premium to Garfield to care for insured workers. Another 12.5% would be used to cover the costs of transferring patients to Los Angeles. The figure of 12.5% was equivalent to $1.50 per worker per month or a nickel (five cents) a day. (We can only speculate what IIE did with the remaining 75% of the workers' premiums.)

The employers also offered a voluntary pay deduction of another nickel a day for non-industrial coverage. Hence the cost to each worker for prepaid comprehensive coverage was a dime a day. With 5000 workers covered by this plan, $500 a day would be generated in prepayment to GCH. Garfield accepted the deal and CGH was back in business.

Contractors General Hospital was not the first prepayment model plan in America.[72] Paul Starr notes several previous examples, including the Boston Dispensary in 1790 and similar schemes in New York, Philadelphia and elsewhere.[76] The Marine Hospital Service offered comprehensive medical coverage to the American Merchant Marine. In 1868 the Central Pacific Railroad offered comprehensive medical care to its employees. In 1891 the consolidated Edison Company of New York established a prepaid medical care program for its workers. In the early 1900s the Endicotte-Johnson Company, a shoe manufacturer in Johnson City New York, and the Standard Oil Company of Baton Rouge, Louisiana established healthcare programs for their employees. In 1908 the United States enacted a workers' compensation law for federal employees. Beginning in 1910 many states also began to enact workers' compensation laws that require employers and employees to contribute to the cost of healthcare insurance for job-related injuries. In 1929 the Department of Water and Power of the City of Los Angeles contracted with the Ross-Loos Medical Group in Los Angeles for prepaid medical coverage for its 12 000 employees and 25 000 dependants. The rising cost of hospitalisation also gave rise to the so-called Blue Cross approach, first developed by Baylor University in Dallas, Texas and formally endorsed by the American Hospital Association in 1933. The Mayo Clinic founded in the 1880s in Rochester, Minnesota was an early prototype of the privately owned group practice.

However, the principles of prepayment and group practice contradicted the dominant model of solo fee-for-service practice in America and were bitterly opposed by many state and county medical societies. Prepaid group practice introduced a third party payer between physician and patient in the form of a health benefit plan. The medical societies thought that this compromised the proper physician–patient relationship, particularly in terms of the patient's free choice of physician, and the physician's professional autonomy. For this reason, the group model remained a minor development in early twentieth-century America.

Garfield faced no such opposition in the Mojave Desert as there were no competing doctors. With prepayment Garfield actually gained his autonomy. Seeing no further need to retain the 12.5% earmarked for Los Angeles Hospitals, IIE increased its contribution to Garfield from 12.5 to 17.5%. Prepayment reversed the normal economics of medicine. The economic incentive to treat liberally was replaced by an incentive to prevent the occurrence or advance of conditions. And whereas fee-for-service patients tended to delay seeking medical help, prepaid members presented early, often helping to prevent more serious outcomes.

When the aqueduct reached the Parker Dam construction site, 125 miles from Desert Centre, Garfield resolved to build another hospital at the Dam site. Parker Dam was being built by a consortium of contractors, called the Six Companies, which include the Henry J Kaiser Company. During its previous construction of the Hoover Dam, the Six Companies had supported a medical care program similar to that provided by Garfield for the Metropolitan Water District, though it excluded voluntary deductions for off-the-job illness and injury cover. Garfield offered the Six Companies a similar program to that provided for the aqueduct workers. It was accepted and Garfield built the Parker Dam Hospital. He built a third hospital at the construction site of Imperial Dam 150 miles south of Parker, part of a Six Companies construction project to irrigate the Imperial Valley in southern California. By 1938, having retained $250 000, Garfield planned to invest in the fee-for-service practice in LA that he had deferred for five years. But it was not to be.

Grand Coulee: 1938–1941

In 1938 the Henry J Kaiser Company was awarded the contract to build the

Coulee Dam in the state of Washington. Garfield was asked to establish a prepaid medical program for Kaiser employees and their dependants at the construction site. Although initially intending to decline the offer, Garfield saw its potential to develop the group model. Unlike the aqueduct project, strung out over 242 miles, the Coulee Dam project was contained on one large site. As in the Mojave Desert, Garfield and his associates believed they could achieve high levels of preventative care at Grand Coulee. Once again they noticed a reduction in the severity of conditions presented by workers and their dependants. They saw acute appendicitis instead of peritonitis, earaches instead of mastoiditis, upper respiratory infections and less pneumonia, early lumps in the breast instead of metastatic carcinoma.

World War II and the shipyards: 1942–1945

In September 1942 Great Britain stood alone against the Axis Powers and depended on shipping convoys from the United States. In that month, the British Admiralty sent a Technical Merchant Shipbuilding Commission to the United States to organise the construction of merchant ships in American shipyards. A commission to build 60 freighters was awarded to the Todd-California Ship-building Consortium organised by Henry J Kaiser and the Todd Shipbuilding Company of Seattle. The Consortium planned to build 30 of the freighters in Richmond on East San Francisco Bay, a few miles north of Oakland.

In December 1941, Japan bombed Pearl Harbor and the United States entered the War. The US Maritime Commission also then became a Kaiser client. Kaiser and others applied assembly line production methods, developed by Henry Ford for car assembly, to shipbuilding. Prefabricated sections travelled on railroad flatcars from throughout the United States to be put together at the shipyards. Eventually the shipyards mounted a competition to see who could build a Liberty ship quickest. Permanente Metals Corporation (Kaiser) No.2 Yard in Richmond, California won the competition. The keel for the SS Robert E. Peary was laid at 12:01 am on 8 November 1942 and 250 000 parts weighing about 14 000 000 pounds were assembled in 4 days, 15 hours and 29 minutes. She was launched on 12 November 1942. At an average cost of $1.8 million, the 'expendable' Liberty ships had to make just one trip to be considered successful.[80]

During the War, Kaiser shipyards delivered 821 Liberty ships (small freighters), 50 small aircraft carriers, 219 Victory-class cargo ships, 24 freighters of other descriptions, 45 troop transports, 87 combat transports, 45 landing ship tank vessels, 12 frigates, and 147 tankers, for a total of more than 15 million deadweight tons of shipping.* By late 1943, about 90 000 men and women worked in the Kaiser shipyards, 30 000 in Richmond. Garfield was again called upon to organise their medical care. By late 1944 he had 90 physicians and staff at three locations: the Richmond yards, the Vancouver-Portland yards on the Columbia River between Washington and Oregon, and the Kaiser steel mill in Fontana, southern California.

---

*These figures are from Smillie who does not quote his source. A full list of the 2751 Liberty ships along with their builders is available from the United States Maritime Marine website: www.usmm.org/libertyships.html.

In 1942 Garfield purchased and renovated the unused Fabiola Hospital at the corner of Broadway and MacArthur in Oakland. The renovated 54-bed facility was called the Permanente Foundation Hospital. *Permanente*, Spanish for permanent, was the name given by Spanish settlers to the Ria Permanente, a stream in the Los Altos Hills of Santa Clara County, south of San Francisco. In the late 1930s, Kaiser had built a cement factory on land watered by the Ria Permanente. He gave its name to the cement works, the medical foundation and several other enterprises, including the Richmond shipyards. By 1945 the Permanente Foundation Hospital had grown to 300 beds and the Richmond Field Hospital from 10 to 100 beds.

Two other prepaid group-practice programs were developing in collaboration with Kaiser Industries. One served the Kaiser shipyards on the Columbia River where it passes between Portland, Oregon and Vancouver, Washington; the other was at the Kaiser steel plant at Fontana, southern California. Although both were under the general supervision of Sidney Garfield, the influence of Ernest Saward in Portland-Oregon, and Raymond Kay in southern California, deserves greater recognition than Smillie's northern Californian perspective perhaps allows. Both men were formidable leaders whose influence extended beyond their own regions and into the whole program at key points in its development.

As in California, 'trainloads of workers began to pour into Portland in early 1942, showing the same walking pathological museum characteristics – pneumonia especially – as their Californian counterparts'.[72] Early in 1942, Edgar Kaiser, one of Henry J Kaiser's two sons and manager at the Portland-Vancouver yards, invited Garfield up to Oregon to establish a comprehensive medical care program for his workers, similar to that established at Richmond. Garfield initially wanted to locate the hospital in Portland, which had 50 000 workers, as against 40 000 in Vancouver. But the medical establishment opposed the idea. The leader of the opposition, Dr Thomas Joyce, was also Edgar Kaiser's personal physician. As Edgar Kaiser accommodated Joyce's views, Garfield was reluctantly obliged to follow. Hence the Northern Permanente Foundation Hospital was built on the Vancouver side of the river, where a combined industrial and non-industrial program was offered to shipyard workers. Portland workers were offered only industrial cover, whilst non-industrial care was provided through a plan involving all Portland physicians. The Hospital opened in June 1942 with 75 beds. It expanded continuously, peaking at 330 beds by the end of 1944.

Whereas the Permanente Medical Foundation at Richmond operated through Sidney Garfield and Associates, the Northern Permanente Foundation was incorporated in 1942 as a non-profit charitable Foundation that operated its medical care program directly. There were other notable differences between the Portland-Vancouver and northern California programs. Whereas in Richmond Garfield recruited a core of physicians, under the strong leadership of Cecil Cutting, who were committed to prepaid group practice, the Portland-Vancouver program suffered an initial lack of both these advantages. Allocation of physicians in the northwest region was controlled by the Seattle Medical Society, which imposed severe restrictions in addition to wartime scarcity. 'I had to go to them to get physicians. I would come up to Seattle and tell them I needed doctors. [...] They were friendly to me. But they'd say, "This guy is no damn good. You take him. We don't care what you do with him." They gave me a couple of good men whom they wanted to keep out of the Army because they liked them so much, and felt they wanted them to remain in the Seattle vicinity. But the majority of men they gave us were men they didn't think were worth much, 4Fs. So we had a group of men at Vancouver who really weren't interested in making our plan work. They weren't producing, and they didn't care about the utilisation of the hospital. We just couldn't make the plan pay.'[79]

To improve the situation at Portland-Oregon, Garfield and Edgar Kaiser contrived in 1943 to get Wally Neighbor released from the Army to become chief executive officer and medical director of the Northern Permanente Foundation. Neighbor, a close friend of Garfield's from his Los Angeles Country General Hospital days, took the Portland-Vancouver program in hand. This experience underlined an important lesson to Garfield: 'No matter how the principles of our plan are meant, if they don't have the physician group who have it in their hearts to make it work and who believe in prepaid practice, it won't work. This is the thing that makes me wonder about HMOs all over the country. They aren't going to work unless they get men in those operations who really believe in giving service to the people.'[79]

It happened that another prepaid group-practice program was operating in the Portland-Oregon area, serving a secret project by the DuPont Company at Hartford in central Washington state. The Hartford project was part of the Manhattan Project to build the atomic bomb. Its medical care program was directed by Ernest Saward, an internist specialising in pulmonary medicine – ideal for the high prevalence of pneumonia among the Kaiser shipyard workers. The Hartford project wound down in 1944. Saward was appointed chief of medicine in Northern Permanente in June 1945. Saward would not only lead the post-war development of the Northern Permanente Foundation program, he would also play a key role in overcoming the problems that beset the early years of the Hawaii Permanente Medical Group, as we shall see later in the section.

There was no foundation in Fontana, where Garfield initially provided medical and hospital services as sole proprietor of what was eventually named the Kaiser Fontana Hospital Association. Raymond Kay served his internship alongside Sidney Garfield and Wally Neighbor at Los Angeles County Hospital. Though Kay and Garfield stayed in touch, they did not work together again until the 1940s. It was Kay who had investigated foundation status, and proposed to Garfield that he should establish a foundation to set aside funds for capital to start a prepaid group practice in Los Angeles after the war. Garfield liked the idea and proposed it to Henry J Kaiser, who concurred. Kaiser's lawyer, Paul Marrin, initially disagreed: how, he objected, could a foundation be formed with only operational income and no capital outlay? Kaiser was not to be deterred, so Marrin took the problem to his partner Robert Bridges, a tax specialist. A few days later, the Permanente Foundation, a charitable trust, was established in Alameda County, California, with Mr and Mrs Henry J Kaiser, Edgar Kaiser, Eugene Trefethan Jr, and a number of their attorneys, acting as trustees.

Kay led the southern California program for many years. He was not afraid to argue with Henry J Kaiser over organisational as well as clinical matters. It was Kay who informed Kaiser that the medical group declined a proposal to rename themselves after him, preferring to retain Permanente in their title. Kaiser reacted petulantly to this rebuff: 'Of course, of course, I wouldn't let him (Kay) use my name. I don't want them to use my name. I wouldn't let them use my name.' 'It is just as if we'd taken candy away from him,' Kay later recalled,[32]

> By late 1944, 100 physicians and their support staff were caring for 200 000 workers and their dependents in northern California, the Pacific Northwest, and southern California. By the spring of 1945, as World War II drew to a close, the program's facilities consisted of the 100-bed Richmond Field Hospital, the 300-bed Permanente Hospital in Oakland, the 330-bed Northern Permanente Hospital in Clark County near Vancouver, and the 60-bed hospital in Fontana. Kaiser Permanente was already the largest civilian prepaid medical program in American history.[72]

Yet within a few months, the shipyards were closed. The 90 000 Richmond workforce shrank to 13 000, and the medical group reduced from 75 to 12 physicians. The need for the Permanente medical program seemed to disappear with the War. Doctors left to take up fee-for-service practice. With dissolution on the agenda and many doctors having already left, the medical staff at Vancouver and northern California met. But, instead of closure, they voted to open the health plan to local communities.

Survival and reorganisation in the post-war era: 1946–1951

In September 1945 a non-profit trust called the Permanente Health Plan was established to take the program into the post-war era. Incorporation was avoided, the connotation of corporate medicine being then taboo in the medical profession. The Health Plan enrolled members and collected dues. The Permanente Foundation still owned the hospitals and carried the debts. Sidney Garfield remained sole proprietor of the medical group and ran the whole program as executive director. He leased the hospitals from the Foundation and all staff were his employees. Despite their differing legal and tax identities, Garfield effectively ran all three entities as an integrated unit. The Plan gained from California's post-war boom. There was plenty of work and most shipyard workers, having enjoyed life in sunny California, did not wish to return to their homes in the east and south.

But opposition to the Permanente Health Plan from medical organisations emerged more strongly after the War. From the perspective of traditional fee-for-service physicians, the special need for prepaid group medicine had gone with the return of hundreds of physicians from military service. In northern California the Alameda-Contra Costa Medical Society criticised the Plan, believing, mistakenly, that the Oakland and Richmond hospitals had been built at taxpayers' expense. It argued that the hospitals be turned over to Alameda County for the care of public charges. The Alameda-Contra Costa Medical Society exploited any advantage. In 1946 Henry J Kaiser started an automobile factory at Willow Run, Michigan. Among the returning veterans considered by Garfield for the post of medical director at Willow Run was Lt Col Clifford Keene, an experienced combat surgeon with extensive operating and medical experience in the Pacific. Preferring California to Michigan, Keene joined the surgical staff at Permanente Hospital, Oakland. Keene did not have a California medical licence, so Garfield appointed him temporary resident, even though Keene had finished his residency in Michigan before the War. This irregularity played into the hands of the Alameda-Contra Costa Medical Society, which complained about Garfield to the California Board of Medical Examiners. After a hearing, the Board suspended Garfield's own medical licence. Garfield contested the suspension in superior court, which overturned the CBME's decision. The CBME then took its case to the appeal court. Meanwhile, Keene took his medical examination for California. Sitting for two gruelling days before his examiners, Keene recalled, 'I believe they were determined that I would fail. But I didn't fail, and I was given a license…They'd ask me a question and I'd write it down and then I'd give them an answer, because I realised that I was being examined by a hostile board.'[73] With the granting of a California licence to Keene, *Garfield v the Board of Medical Examiners* was dropped. The Alameda-Contra Costa Medical Society found other occasions to attack Garfield and his medical group, including accusing him of advertising and soliciting patients for the Health Plan.

In the immediate post-war years, Garfield struggled to keep the program going on its 10 000 membership. Increasing membership, in order to increase operating revenue and generate capital for investment, was hindered by a ban on promoting medical services. At this time most employers did not provide health insurance for their employees. When they did, a favourable group premium rate required at least 75% of employees to be covered by a single plan. In the mid-1940s, Blue Cross and California Physicians Service (Blue Shield) were the two major plans. Some unions were wary of associating with Kaiser as a major industrialist, which worked against the Permanente Health Plan. Moreover, politically conservative unions and employer groups were wary of prepaid group medical care as 'socialised medicine', a phrase still used by some Americans to denigrate Kaiser Permanente and other HMOs. Many San Francisco Bay Area residents assumed the Permanente Plan to be still limited to Kaiser employees, whom some regarded as shipyard riff-raff, not understanding that subscription was open to the public. Hence, the program was regarded as inferior by many people at different points on the political compass, which certainly did not help it to survive and flourish.

In February 1948 the program was restructured into the Permanente Health Plan, Permanente Hospitals, and the Permanente Medical Group. The Health Plan continued as a non-profit trust, governed by lay trustees. The Permanente Hospitals and the Permanente Medical Group were new entities. The Permanente Foundation and the Northern Permanente Foundation in the Oregon-Washington region continued to own hospitals that Permanente Hospitals ran. The Permanente physicians could not be expected to continue indefinitely in their dependent status as Garfield's employees. On 21 February 1948, the Permanente Medical Group was formally established as a partnership, with seven original partners, including Garfield. On 10 April 1948 the partners determined that there should be three categories in the Group: senior partners, junior partners, and physician employees. On 1 July 1949 Garfield withdrew from the partnership of the group he had founded. As senior officer of the Health Plan and the Hospitals, he was administering a charitable corporation and a non-profit trust, respectively. This dual role sat uncomfortably with his role in a profit-making partnership.

Membership rose from a baseline of 10 000 members in mid-1945, to 72 000 by April 1948. Permanente medical care was affordable, consistent and efficient, with all facilities at one location. Universities and civil service organisations, anxious to establish healthcare provision for their members, were among the first attracted to Permanente after the war.

In 1947 the United Steelworkers of America union chose Permanente as an alternative plan and asked companies employing the union's members to provide payroll deductions. The companies refused. In arbitration it was determined that the employers must offer health insurance payment by payroll deduction even when the group health plan was unilaterally selected by the union. This decision strengthened the right of working men and women to select their own healthcare programs.

In 1948 another dispute arose. The Health Service System of the city and county of San Francisco chose to offer Permanente as an alternative choice for city employees. The Retirement Board refused on the grounds that the patient's choice of physician was restricted to Permanente physicians. The Health Service sued the Retirement Board. The California Supreme Court ruling upheld the principle of dual choice, meaning that a choice must be made available between Permanente and a program allowing individual choice of physicians. As a result, dual choice was adopted as a key principle of the Permanente Health Plan. Permanente physicians were adamant that no one should be forced to join Permanente: there should always be an alternative. This would help to avoid resentment by patients who perceived a lack of choice.

Also in 1948, civilian workers at Hunters Point Naval Shipyard enrolled in the program. This led the Permanente Foundation to purchase a 35-bed hospital near the Shipyard, at 331 Pennsylvania Street in San Francisco's Bayshore District.

In 1945 the tenant council of Vallejo Housing Authority asked Permanente to establish a medical centre for tenants and employees in Vallejo, on the northern San Francisco Bay. The Vallejo program increased rapidly from 500 members in 1945 to 30 000 in 1954, by which time a Permanente clinic in Napa also served 5 000 members.

In 1950 the International Longshoremen and Warehousemen Union, and the Retail Clerks union in Los Angeles brought Permanente to southern California. The ILWU membership required the establishment of Health Plan cover along the entire Pacific coast from Seattle to San Diego. Consequently, new Permanente Plans were located in Seattle, Los Angeles and San Diego. As Seattle already had a prepaid group practice plan, the Group Health Cooperative of Puget Sound, Garfield arranged for Group Health to take the ILWU contract up there. The health needs of ILWU members in the San Francisco Bay Area were covered by existing Oakland, San Francisco, Richmond and Vallejo facilities. However, the inland port of Stockton on the San Joaquin River presented a challenge, being 60 miles east of Oakland. Permanente was not keen to establish a plan that far from its major hospitals. The solution was found when a group of Stockton physicians established the San Joaquin Foundation for Medical Care, a prepaid plan. Hospitalisation was subcontracted to the Pacific National Life Insurance Company. In San Diego a similar arrangement was made for a small existing health plan to take care of the longshoremen. In Los Angeles, the ILWU contract required a new hospital, as the 60-bed Fontana hospital was 45 miles away. Initially an arrangement was made to admit southern California Permanente Health Plan patients to a local hospital. The Foundation rented space in a medical office building in San Pedro and established a clinic there. But opposition by the Wilmington-San Pedro medical community persuaded the fee-for-service clinicians who owned the building to evict the Permanente physicians.

New accommodation was found a week before eviction. That experience reinforced one of the ground rules of the Permanente program: ownership and integration of hospital facilities. It could not afford to risk dependency on the goodwill and cooperation of uncommitted parties. 'For the Permanente program to function properly, hospital, clinic, office space, and laboratory had to be in a single or adjacent buildings under Permanente ownership where all medical services could take place. Not only was such an arrangement more efficient; it also protected Permanente from outside interference or, in some cases, outright harassment by a hostile medical community.'[72] Seven months later, Garfield was approached by the Retail Clerks Union in Los Angeles, which sought a comprehensive healthcare program for its 30 000 members. In 1951 the RCU joined Permanente, leading to the establishment of a second Los Angeles clinic in the Rexall Building on La Cienega Boulevard. In February 1953 Permanente built and opened the first phase of the 200-bed Sunset Hospital in Los Angeles.

When the Columbia River shipyards closed at the end of the war, the Northern Permanente Health Plan did not rebound with the same vigour as the San Francisco Bay Area. Three miles from Vancouver, the hospital was inconveniently located for the civilian population. Portland residents were reluctant to join a program on the Washington side of the river; nor did they want their babies born in a different state. In 1945 membership was 15 000. In April 1946 it dropped to 3 000. It grew only slowly, reaching 14 000 in 1950 and 23 000 in 1953.

As in the Bay Area, the local medical community was generally hostile. In 1945 the Washington State Medical Society declared that the Northern Permanente Foundation was unethical. Saward, the only Permanente physician member of the WSMS, appealed to the AMA Judicial Council. The charge was withdrawn in 1946. Even so, the employment of physicians by the Foundation, a lay organisation, remained a sticking point, which the Northern Permanente physicians removed by forming a medical group partnership, The Permanente Clinic, in late 1946.

On top of these obstacles, Vanport Hospital, acquired by the Northern Permanente Foundation in 1947, was swept away by a flood in May 1948. It was empty at the time.

The struggle for control: 1952–1955

By August 1952 Permanente was serving 250 000 members, 160 000 of them in northern California. One hundred and twenty five physicians were practising with the Permanente Medical Group. The Permanente Hospitals were operating four facilities with a total bed capacity of 500. Clinics were operating in Walnut Creek, Redwood City, and Napa. Three major hospitals were in planning or construction: one in Los Angeles (built on a part of Barnsdall Park), one in San Francisco (on Geary Boulevard, near Divisadero), and one in Walnut Creek. The Permanente Hospitals maintained a successful nursing school and an intern and resident training program. $250 000 was allocated to research including the acquisition of a research laboratory in Belmont.

But by 1952 a power struggle had grown between Kaiser and the doctors for control over the Permanente program. The relationship between Henry J Kaiser and Sidney Garfield was complex. Garfield was and always remained Kaiser's personal physician. Garfield was also personal physician to Kaiser's first wife, Bess, until she died of chronic nephritis. For her final six months, the Garfields lived with the Kaisers in their penthouse on Lake Merritt in Oakland. Garfield moved a Permanente nurse, Alyce Chester, into the Kaiser apartment to look after Mrs Kaiser, who died on 15 March 1951. On 10 June 1951 Henry J Kaiser aged 69 married Alyce Chester aged 34. Less than a year later, Sidney Garfield had divorced his first wife, Virginia, and married Alyce's sister Helen. The Garfields moved next door to the Kaisers in Lafayette. Garfield and Kaiser, now brothers-in-law, were frequently in and out of each other's homes. Previously content to let Garfield run the Permanente program, after his marriage to Alyce, Kaiser became increasingly involved in its affairs. This coincided with a protracted period of conflict between Kaiser and the physicians. This was an important episode in the history of the program because Kaiser 'began to try to control the program, including its physicians. Kaiser's energy, vision, will, and obsession with growth and construction, and his new and compelling interest in medicine as he understood it, brought him into a decade-long conflict with the same physicians whose medical care program he had supported in the previous decade with a minimum of interference. The stage was set for a titanic battle of wills.'[72] The main casualty of the battle was Garfield himself.

Having married a young nurse, Kaiser decided to build her a hospital in Walnut Creek, a community in a warm valley 20 miles east of Oakland. This was controversial to the doctors for several reasons. It was unilateral on Kaiser's part. It involved what they saw as a misappropriation of funds. The funds in dispute had been set aside by the Medical Group during the lean post-war years to commit to major hospitals in Los Angeles and San Francisco. As well as being open to Health Plan members, Kaiser's new showcase Walnut Creek hospital would be available to fee-for-service physicians. 'Kaiser was using revenues – some of which were generated by Permanente physicians – to subsidise a luxury hospital for fee-for-service physicians in the Walnut Creek area. It was a bitter pill for Permanente physicians to swallow.'[72] Not only was the Permanente Medical Group not consulted about the Walnut Creek hospital, it was ignored about staffing it, too. Remarkably, Alyce Chester personally selected the medical staff on her own authority.*

In 1952 the Health Plan and the Hospitals formally adopted the name *Kaiser*. From that point the program comprised the Kaiser Foundation Health Plan and the Kaiser Foundation Hospitals. The Permanente Medical Group, however, refused to change its name to Kaiser Medical Group. The reason given was that such a name would imply that they were employees of Henry J Kaiser and not an autonomous medical partnership. But the refusal also reflected the physicians' resentment over the Walnut Creek hospital. Kaiser responded to the refusal aggressively, proposing that the Medical Group be divided into smaller separate partnerships. In the background he had articles of incorporation prepared for a separate Walnut Creek medical group that he and Alyce could control. His

---

*In retrospect, Kaiser correctly anticipated the growth of the Concord-Walnut Creek area where, by the late 1980s, there would be 300 000 Health Plan members, compared with 5000 in 1952.

divide-and-conquer strategy failed, however, the Walnut Creek physicians refused to form a separate Group and joined the Permanente Medical Group.

As an advocate of the Walnut Creek hospital, Garfield found himself caught between Kaiser and the doctors. He had also tried to convince the Medical Group to change its name to Kaiser. Moreover, during the height of the McCarthy witch-hunts, on the order of the Kaiser organisation, Garfield became involved in firing three physicians suspected of being Communists.

By 1952 several major issues had emerged between The Kaiser Foundation/ Hospitals/Health Plan and the Permanente Medical Group. Most contentious was the question of who *owned* the program. Physicians identified the program with their medical practice and considered the Kaiser Health Plan as an agency to enrol patients and collect dues. They saw the Kaiser Foundation Hospitals as their workshops. Seeing themselves as revenue generators of the program, the doctors thought they should be in control. Kaiser Industries took a different view. They saw the Foundation and the Health Plan as leading the program. Members belonged to the Plan, not to the Medical Group, which serviced the Plan members' needs. As members were the source of their income, the Plan, not the physicians, was clearly the income generating entity. Furthermore, the Foundation and the Plan had capital in the Hospitals and carried the indebtedness, whereas the doctors only practised medicine. Finally, medics had no claim to govern and administer the program: these were clearly responsibilities of businesspeople.

The history of Kaiser Permanente up to that point supported both perspectives. Garfield and the Medical Group had founded and developed the program from an identified need for occupational healthcare in the Mojave Desert to a multimillion dollar turnover business. On the other hand, they had achieved this only with the material support, personal sponsorship and credit rating of Kaiser. In fact the claims appear more or less even: without the Plan and Hospitals there would be no Medical Group, and vice versa. The program's unique financial structure, operation and ethos were owed equally to Kaiser and the doctors, even after it was opened to non-Kaiser employees.

The conflict was brought into the open by Henry J Kaiser's unilateral allocation of funds, in part saved by the Medical Group, to his and Alyce's pet Walnut Creek project; and the trappings of luxury incompatible with the Medical Group's prudential ethos. It came down to money. Medical Group compensation was inconsistent, being subject to periodic alteration to account for the growing program's expenses. There were also surcharges for certain services. For example, flat fees were charged for registration, maternity care, tonsillectomies, laboratory and X-ray services. These were collected and retained by Kaiser Hospitals though physicians held that they should have been returned to the Medical Group.

These chronic tensions came to a head in 1955 after the Walnut Creek development. The Kaiser camp declared that the Kaiser organisation ran whatever it was involved in. The Medical Group disputed that claim on the basis that medical care was qualitatively different from dams, ships, steel and cement. The doctors were also concerned that they still did not even have a retirement plan. And there was a question mark over the fate of the Retention Fund, accumulated by contributions from their earnings to cover their contractual commitments in the event of financial failure. With that danger fading, what would happen to that money now?

In early 1954 the Medical Group Executive Committee had proposed three alternative futures for the program. First, the physicians could give up their independence and become employees of the Health Plan. Second, separate partnerships could be organised at each facility. Third, the Medical Group partnership could stay intact but with a new emphasis on the regions in which the major medical care centres were located. In June 1954 the Executive Committee recommended the third option: the Health Plan and Hospitals would remain under central control but would also be diversified in regional administrative units working alongside the already diversified physician groups in the form of the northern California, southern California and Oregon-Washington partnerships. But first this semi-devolved confederation had to gain the approval of trustees, administrators and physicians.

By April 1955 dissent between stakeholders had reached crisis level and organisational paralysis had set in. 'Expansion was stopped, membership was stopped, spending of money was stopped, everything ground to a halt.'[13] On April 21, in a joint letter to Eugene Trefethen, a trustee of the Kaiser Foundation and Kaiser's right-hand-man, the regional medical groups proposed the formation of a working council to deal with the impasse: 'We consider the basic problems to be the obtaining of a mutually satisfactory integration of all managerial activities, mutually satisfactory representation at policy-making levels, mutually satisfactory methods of monetary distribution and control, and mutually satisfactory methods of selection of all key personnel.' The pounding repetition of 'mutually satisfactory' effectively conveys the extent of dissatisfaction felt by physicians concerning the status quo.

The committee was duly formed and met on four occasions with varying degrees of success and conflict. At the first meeting, on 12–13 May 1955, the Medical Group tabled five possible future scenarios. The medical groups could take over the entire operation including the Health Plan (option 1) and the Hospitals (option 2). The medical groups could be given equal representation on the boards of trustees of the Health Plan or the Hospitals or both (option 3). The differences could be resolved by contractual agreements between the medical groups and the Health Plan (option 4). Or (option 5) the situation could remain as it was: the trustees being responsible for the management of Health Plan and Hospitals; the medical groups responsible for medical care.

Option 4 – contractual arrangements between the medical groups and the Health Plan – contained the germ of a long-term solution. In hindsight it is amazing that the program could have continued to operate so long without such arrangements. That it had done so and thrived was due in large part to the energy and influence of Sidney Garfield, whose role had by then been marginalised. In fact, the contractual option was not immediately appealing to the working council. Kaiser attorney George Link was directed to consider the tax consequences of all five proposals. His report was compelling, as we shall see.

The Committee's second meeting, on 7 June 1955, was less constructive, partly as Henry J Kaiser attended along with Henry J Kaiser Jr, and a formidable array of Kaiser executives. Kaiser himself opened the meeting by proposing that the trustees withdraw completely and permit the doctors to manage the program through small independent groups. This suggestion was unhelpful and irrelevant in the light of Link's report on the tax implications of the five options floated at the first meeting. Everybody present already knew that a physician buy-out was impossible. Any change in ownership or governance would jeopardise the Kaiser Foundation Hospitals' tax-exempt status. If the Medical Group, a for-profit enterprise, took over the hospitals, Kaiser Foundation Hospitals would become liable for additional property, payroll, rental and income taxes from its operation totalling about $4 339 600 for the period 1 January 1955 to 31 December 1959. If, as in option 3, the component organisations remained under Kaiser ownership, but doctors were allowed equal representation on all boards, that too would endanger the tax-exempt status of the Foundation Hospitals, incurring a demand for back taxes in excess of $2m plus interest. Such a lump sum obligation would bankrupt both the Kaiser Foundation and Kaiser Foundation Hospitals. Should the Medical Group choose to purchase the Kaiser Foundation Hospitals, their book value as of December 1954 was $15 416 000, less mortgages totalling $6 225 000, giving a net cash price of $9 200 000. As Smillie comments, such stark financial considerations 'grounded all further discussion in reality. Whatever their objections to lay control might be, the physicians had to recognise that the present set-up had allowed a significant portion of the program tax-exempt status. Without such tax exemptions, the Kaiser-Permanente program – and hence the physicians' personal incomes – could not have flourished. The physicians could not have it both ways. If they chose to own and operate the program, or even to serve on the board of trustees, they would have to assume the financial consequences.'[72] Link considered the fourth option the most feasible. Contractual agreements were the only realistic solution to the impasse.

Perhaps fortunately, Kaiser did not attend the third meeting on 21–22 June 1955, though the first afternoon was still wasted discussing his futile proposal from the second meeting. On the second day, however, several significant compromises were agreed. A joint Kaiser-Permanente Advisory Committee would be formed to coordinate the program and review appointments of key personnel. Both sides stated their goals and objectives. The question of how to integrate the daily management of the program was considered, for it was in the pragmatic day-to-day administration that authority and responsibility had to be shared between the physicians and administrators. Subcommittees in northern and southern California were appointed to work out a teamwork approach and report back to the final session scheduled for 12 July 1955.

The Tahoe Agreement: 1955–1960

The fourth and final session of the working council to consider the future of the Kaiser Permanente program convened at Henry J Kaiser's *Fleur de Lac* estate on Lake Tahoe. As well as being a watershed in the history of Kaiser Permanente, the Lake Tahoe conference and the Tahoe Agreement it produced have entered the institution's folklore. At Tahoe Sidney Garfield was finally removed from the line of authority. At Tahoe Henry J Kaiser came face-to-face with a collective will among physicians as strong as his own. They were not prepared to become his employees and surrender their autonomy. But it was at Tahoe too that many of the same physicians realised the necessity to give up any idea of buying out Kaiser to take ownership of the hospitals and the Health Plan. No minutes were taken of the Tahoe Conference.[72] The previous day, Kaiser had asked, then ordered, Garfield to resign. Confident he would be supported by the Medical Group, Garfield agreed to resign if the Medical Group approved. It did. 'I didn't think they would,' Garfield admitted. 'When [Kaiser] met with them the next day, they accepted it immediately. I felt let down. After that, my job was planning and building facilities.'[2]

After three days of discussion, the meeting resulted in a document dated 19 July 1955, subsequently known as the Tahoe Agreement. It contained six resolutions. First, a commitment from all parties to preserve the medical care program and to find a way for all entities to work together to that end. Second, an advisory council was permanently established comprising representatives of the medical groups, Health Plan and Hospitals. Third, to create regional executive management teams comprising the regional Health Plan Manager, the Hospital Manager, and the key physician administrators of each region. Fourth, all problem areas would be covered by the contracts between medical groups and the Health Plan. Those areas would include the approval of Health Plan contracts, the question of advertising and/or solicitation of new members, the establishment of continuity of control with the Health Plan, and the assurance that the Health Plan would not develop competing groups in the regions. Fifth, financial arrangements were agreed whereby the Hospitals and the medical groups would be supported in their basic needs, and excess revenue would be equally distributed. Sixth, Permanente Services would be established as a service organisation supporting all entities. (Permanente Services eventually provided a wide range of services including accounting, purchasing, warehousing, data processing, employee and community relations, planning services and facilities management.)

The regional management teams were established to mediate between regional personnel and the national advisory council; and to coordinate and review all activities within the region of the Health Plan, the Hospitals, and Permanente Services. The regional management teams were not intended to merge or amalgamate existing administrative structures. Each of the regional Health Plans, Hospitals and medical groups retained its authority and responsibilities.

The Tahoe Conference also created a third level of administration called area management teams. They comprised the physician-in-chief or associate medical director of each area, and the local hospital administrator. It was also agreed that neither party could take any action that might affect the other, without prior mutual consultation.

The Tahoe Conference did not end all conflict between Kaiser and Permanente, but it did clarify and affirm the important relationship between physicians and managers in the organisation and delivery of healthcare, and placed the medical groups on a firmer financial footing. As Smillie reflects, 'It would take a few more tumultuous years for this newly asserted mutuality of respect to solidify itself as a permanent feature of the Kaiser-Permanente corporate culture. Perceived in retrospect as a watershed, as a near legendary battle of giants, the Tahoe Conference and the subsequent agreement set the stage for the more viable solutions and the more lasting agreements that were to come.'[72]

In fact the advisory council was not permanent and met only seven times between August 1955 and June 1956. During this time, however, contracts were agreed between Kaiser Health Plan and Permanente Medical Groups. Termed

Medical Service Agreements, these contracts helped to carry the program into a new era. They covered the following eight policy areas, which still serve to define the character of the Kaiser Permanente program to the present day.

1   *Per capita contracting:* Previously, contracts between the Health Plan and medical groups had been based on a somewhat variable percentage of pre-paid dues. The proposed payment would be based on a mutually agreed upon per capita rate. This way, revenue was more closely tied to actual operating experience.
2   *Minimum capital generation requirement:* To protect its financial stability the group must generate revenues to meet its per capita costs and straight line depreciation plus 4% of the historical cost of land, building, and equipment. Such obligations constituted the minimum consistent with long-term financial self-sufficiency.
3   *Incentive compensation:* Revenues in excess of those required under the minimum capital generation requirement were to be divided equally between the medical groups and the Hospitals. This would satisfy the partnership concept, act as a financial incentive for physicians, and serve as a means to increase Hospital earnings from the minimum to adequate levels.
4   *The program revenue concept:* Revenue from all sources should be combined into a single total of revenue available to support all operations of the program. For legal and ethical reasons, only revenue from house calls was exempted and belonged exclusively to the medical groups.
5   *Regional financial autonomy:* Each region should be considered financially autonomous in terms of revenue and accountability.
6   *Simplified organisational structure:* The Kaiser Foundation, having donated all facilities to Kaiser Foundation Hospitals, should relinquish any remaining ownership or holding function. Henceforth, there would be only three major program entities: The Health Plan, the Hospitals and the medical groups.
7   *Joint management concept:* The regional management teams were not working and should be abandoned. The partnership concept, however, must remain intact. There should therefore be a joint medical director–regional manager structure. The medical director would be the chief executive of the medical group. The regional manager would be the chief executive of the Hospitals and Health Plan in the region. As well as being responsible for their respective organisations, they would be jointly responsible for the effective functioning of the total program in the region.
8   *Physicians' retirement plan:* Though the program had been running for 15 years, it had no retirement provision for physicians. This should be explored.

Regional management teams

The regional management teams differed considerably in constitution and practice. Actually, no regional management team was established in Oregon-Washington. The Permanente Clinic in Oregon continued under its existing arrangements, with Ernest Saward dominating the decision-making process in the North West region. Saward, medical director of the Permanente Clinic in Oregon, also became the de facto chief executive officer for the Health Plan and the Hospitals. No objections to this were raised by the trustees at the Tahoe Conference.* In northern California, a complete regional management team was appointed, with Morris Collen and Cecil Cutting representing The Permanente Medical Group, LeMonte Baritell representing Permanente Services, Hal Babbet representing the Health Plan, and Felix Day representing the Hospitals. A doctor rotated as chairperson every six months.

Overall, it seems that southern California was the most moderate region in terms of their relations between the different constituencies of the program: 'Despite the confrontational style of Ray Kay, relations between the physicians, the Health Plan, and the Hospitals in southern California were actually functioning more cordially than in the north. Ray Kay and Karl Steil were already working out a de facto joint management structure.† Southern California was also in a period of major growth and was hence doubly anxious to achieve arrangements that would allow it to get on with the business of providing prepaid comprehensive healthcare to a rapidly expanding southland.'[72]

To grasp the full significance of this aspiration, one has to appreciate the dynamic social and economic conditions of southern California in the 1930s. Tens of thousands of those whom the press called Dust Bowl refugees settled in southern California. They came from the southern plains states of Oklahoma, Texas, Arkansas, and Missouri. Victims of drought and depression, they headed west hoping for a brighter future in the semi-mythical land of California.[25] Some worked as cotton pickers in the Imperial Valley, watered by the Imperial Dam, constructed by the Six Companies (including Kaiser), where Garfield built his third desert hospital in the late 1930s. Some found even greater material and social hardship in California than they had left behind. Low wages, discrimination and homesickness drove many back to their home states, some to return again.

'After six years of struggle between physicians and the Kaiser organisation, the entire Kaiser-Permanente community had grown weary of infighting.'[72] On 27 March 1958, the executive committee of the Permanente Medical Group approved Medical Service Agreement 1958, which established a framework or constitution for the Kaiser Foundation Health Plan and the Permanente Medical Group which has lasted to this day. Among other things, MSA 1958 stated that the Health Plan would contract exclusively with the Permanente Medical Group so long as the group adequately served the needs of the Health Plan and the membership. Reciprocally, the Medical Group would contract exclusively with the Health Plan and not render professional services to any other prepayment plan in the area.

Between 1955 and 1960 Health Plan membership in northern California grew from 301 000 to 399 000.[72]‡ This rapid growth presented a challenge to physician

---

*Saward also played an important role in helping to establish the Ohio Permanente Medical Group. In 1964 Saward went out to Cleveland and organised several physicians on the Case Western Reserve into a medical group. In 1967 he stepped in again to help facilitate a merger between the Community Health Foundation of Cleveland and the Kaiser Permanente Health Plan to form the Kaiser Community Health Foundation.

†At the Tahoe Conference Kay again came head-to-head with Kaiser. Smillie's account of the incident is telling not only regarding Kay's ability as a forceful defender of medical group autonomy, but also to underline the independent attitude of the Southern California Medical Group. '"You are challenging me," Kaiser exploded at one point to Ray Kay, the feisty head of the Southern California Medical Group. "You're challenging me and I won't stand for it."'

‡Smillie is inconsistent on this point. On p. 159 he puts the figure at only 365 000.

recruitment and deployment. Continuing medical society hostility did not help the situation. The Solano County Medical Society denied membership to Permanente physicians in Vallejo. The San Francisco Medical Society admitted few Permanente physicians, although dialogue was by then improving the situation. In Oakland, Richmond, and Walnut Creek, by contrast, Permanente physicians were increasingly accepted into the medical community. Once ideologically opposed to the prepayment group model, the Alameda-Contra Costa Medical Society now had Permanente physicians serving on its committees. But even members of non-hostile medical societies continued to advise physicians against joining the Permanente Medical Group. In Washington DC the District of Columbia Medical Society and the American Medical Association were found to be in violation of the Sherman Anti-Trust Act by denying membership to physicians associated with the Group Health association, a consumer-owned and sponsored prepaid group-practice plan. The Supreme Court upheld the decision and similar decisions were handed down in Seattle and San Diego.

Friction between Permanente physicians and the Health Plan continued even after Medical Service Agreement 1958, partly due to the Health Plan's failure to consult physicians about certain key appointments. A series of conferences was held between 1958 and 1960 to improve relations between the two entities. The Feather River Inn conference in Autumn 1958 took the form of an encounter group mediated by three professors with expertise in group dynamics, one each from Berkeley, Stanford and UCLA. According to Smillie, the process was 'disorderly and acrimonious…angry invectives being hurled even during coffee breaks and meals. The academic visitors never succeeded in directing the conference into positive channels. When the participants rode by bus back to Oakland on the Sunday afternoon, the atmosphere was subdued.'[72]

The second conference was held in 1959 in Santa Rosa. While not as acrimonious as the Feather River Inn debacle, it achieved little. In May 1960 the first inter-regional management conference was held in Monterey. At that conference Sidney Garfield, who had just been appointed to the board of directors of the Health Plan, urged Kaiser Permanente to alter its strategy away from a traditional focus on treatment, towards the prevention of illness and the maintenance of health. Garfield's appointment to the board was important. It returned the physician founder to a position of power and authority in the core of the program. Garfield's argument was that it should be a health plan, not a sickness plan: committed to maintaining the health of its membership. This ethos continues to resonate in debates on healthcare in the United States, the United Kingdom, and elsewhere, and came to be enshrined in the Health Maintenance Act 1973.

Kaiser Permanente in Hawaii

Hawaiian territories were formally transferred to the United States on 12 August 1898 (with Sanford B Dole as first Governor). Hawaii was admitted to statehood on 21 August 1959, when it became the 50th state in the Union. In 1956, at 75, Henry J Kaiser retired from active direction of the Kaiser companies and moved to Hawaii with his second wife Alyce. Kaiser's arrival was a fateful event for the main administrative island of Oahu, and the city of Honolulu in particular. He saw in Honolulu the potential to develop a major tourist and convention destination similar to Miami, Florida, whose rise he had witnessed as a young man. Kaiser determined that he would be that social planner and developer.

Kaiser's first project was the Hawaiian Village Complex bordering Waikiki Beach, Honolulu. The Complex comprised a 100-room hotel, 70 adjacent thatched-roof cottages, a 1000-seat auditorium, and a 14-story residential tower. By October 1960, when *TIME* magazine profiled Kaiser's Hawaiian empire, he had completed 1600 hotel rooms, together with massive convention facilities. To supply this construction frenzy, Kaiser opened a Permanente cement plant with an annual capacity of 1.7 million barrels. He also entered radio and television broadcasting, the tour boat business, and residential development in Hawaii-Kai, a new community whose predominant feature was Kaiser's favourite pink concrete. Whether Kaiser was a blessing or a curse to Honolulu is perhaps meaningless to pose out of the context of the times. It was perhaps fortunate, however, that he was at least semi-retired. It seems that he was not much interested in planning regulations.

Kaiser took it upon himself to create a health plan that he could run directly, without the interference of the Permanente Medical Group. As at Walnut Creek, he began by constructing a hospital, even though a previous study by Stanford Research Institute had shown that Honolulu had no need of another hospital and that a local medical insurance plan, the Hawaii Medical Services Association, was adequately meeting local needs. Even so, in January 1958 Kaiser began constructing a hospital on Waikiki Beach near to the Hawaiian Village hotel even before he had been granted approval by the Hawaiian authorities. He had decided to sheath the hospital with layers of lava rock, which the city building code specifically barred as it created crawling spaces for rats. Kaiser had the first two floors sheathed in lava before the planners could protest. With typical alacrity the hospital was completed in 10 months.

Kaiser also personally recruited the medical staff. Among Henry and Alyce's social group were three prominent Honolulu physicians, each in solo fee-for-service practice. Kaiser persuaded them to form a partnership practice to establish a medical program at his new hospital. Kaiser was warned by his advisor, Eugene Trefethen, that a Caucasian-only partnership would fail in multi-ethnic Hawaii. Hence Kaiser also recruited two additional prominent physicians, one of Chinese and one of Japanese origin. The Hawaiian partnership called itself Pacific Medical Associates. Kaiser called on one Permanente Group physician and two Kaiser central office staff to help set up the program. In summer 1958 Clifford Keene and Scott Fleming ran crash courses on the medical and financial aspects of prepaid group practice.

But Health Plan enrolment in Hawaii was disappointing. Needing 15 000 to 16 000 members to be financially viable, it opened with only 5000. The Asian communities of the Honolulu area had strong, conservative attachments to their fee-for-service physicians, many of them associated with the established Hawaii Medical Services Association plan. Kaiser Permanente's post-war expansion on the US mainland had been supported by an extensive unionised workforce along the west coast. With the exceptions of the ILWU and the Hotel and Restaurant Workers Union, the Honolulu area did not support an extensive unionised workforce. By mid-1960, enrolment had reached 35 000 but was still insufficient to cover the costs of the Honolulu Medical Centre and the 33 physicians employed by PMA.

This was not the scenario painted by Kaiser for the original five PMA partners, who became increasingly disgruntled. The partners were entitled to continue fee-for-service practice. This violated a basic premise of prepaid group practice. Complaints were made that the wealthy fee-for-service patients (often visitors to Hawaii) received preferential treatment, whilst the prepaid Health Plan patients (the locals) received inferior service. The PMA partners were also shunned by their fee-for-service peers. As Smillie describes, the physicians and their wives were not prepared for the professional and social ostracism they soon experienced: 'This was especially difficult for the wives of a number of the founding partners, who prior to joining Kaiser had enjoyed social prominence in Honolulu. Suddenly, the physicians found themselves cold-shouldered by the local medical society. Physicians and wives alike found themselves increasingly excluded from the social life of the fee-for-service medical community. "They ostracised them to the point that they were just blackballed," recalled Lambreth Hancock, Hawaii Kaiser Health Plan regional manager. "From everything. Their wives, who had been very close to one another – played bridge, played golf, all that sort of thing, in each other's homes all the time for dinner – whoosh, one wife wouldn't speak to the other wife. I mean, it was just a cold-blooded freeze-out."'[74]

In mid-1959 Hancock began to keep a confidential diary of events in the Hawaii region. It detailed a progressive deterioration in relations between the PMA partners and the Kaiser organisation. Kaiser began to call Clifford Keene over to Honolulu frequently to monitor the situation. Trefethen and Keene arranged for Ernest Saward, director of the Kaiser Permanente program in Portland Oregon, to spend the month of April 1960 with PMA. Ostensibly a visiting practitioner at the Honolulu Medical Centre, Saward was actually Trefethen's spy. Many of the associate physicians felt they were being unfairly exploited by the PMA partners, and confided their grievances to Saward. Highly experienced, Saward formed his own assessment of all the medical staff.

In summer 1960 the situation in Hawaii came to a head. The five partners broke contract by demanding immediate increases in compensation from the Health Plan – 'Or else.' The following day, Saturday 20 August, on his own initiative and with only conditional support from Henry J Kaiser ('Clifford, you're all on your own. If you come a cropper on this, you're just out the back door. You'll lose everything.'[73]) Keene sacked the PMA partners, serving them with a written notice to vacate the premises by 5:30pm that day. The remaining 33 employed physicians were assembled and invited to continue to practise as a medical group. All but two stayed. Then Saward and a crack Kaiser team flew over to deal with the embittered ex-partners and reorganise the medical group. Keene appointed himself regional manager over Hancock. Keene and Saward chose Philip Chu, a Chinese-American surgeon on the PMA staff, to be director of the Hawaii Permanente Medical Group. Under Saward's guidance, Hawaii developed a strong, one-person directorship under Chu, as Oregon had done under Saward himself.

The sacked PMA partners tried to wage a public relations war against Henry J Kaiser. But as Kaiser owned a TV and radio station, and controlled a PR setup in his own empire, they were heavily outgunned. After five days a truce was called. The ex-partners took their case to court, claiming major damages for breach of contract. The Kaiser Permanente Health Plan eventually agreed to a token out-of-court settlement.

It took another five years to get the Hawaii Kaiser Permanente program on its feet. In 1969 the Hawaii region expanded to the island of Maui. According to Garfield, the whole Hawaii experience reaffirmed his conviction that not just any physician, however competent, could make the transition to prepaid group practice.[72] After Hawaii, great care was taken in selecting the core cadre for any new medical group. Indeed, as the present study found, every physician recruited to Hawaii Permanente Medical Group has to pass what some regard as the most rigorous selection criterion: Would I want this person to treat my own family? That test has a special significance for the Hawaiian concept of society as potentially one great family. The prominent Hawaiian family ethos (*ohana*) suggests how intolerable social ostracism may have been for the PMA partners. Whereas on the mainland Kaiser Permanente endured the ostracism of some medical societies by virtue of owning its own hospitals, that structural advantage may not have been sufficient to prevent the PMA partners from deserting the program.

We are accustomed to analysing society into separate institutions. For many Hawaii residents who have retained or adopted aspects of Native Hawaiian culture, such an analysis is foreign and untenable. Hawaii is one of the most culturally diverse places in the world. Its amalgam of Native Hawaiian, Polynesian, Asian, and European cultures retains and blends elements of each. Yet as a Pacific culture evolving on one of the most remote island chains in the world (2000 miles from landfall) it retains some unique features. This is obvious from everyday interactions and was made explicit by respondents. At some point in every interview, the respondent would say something like: 'In order to really understand what happened here, you need to understand Hawaiians and their culture.' From Clifford Keene's perspective, Hawaii underlined the necessity for close cooperation and a close community of sentiment between the Health Plan Hospitals and the physicians. Hawaii was difficult, Keene later admitted, but in the long run it strengthened the entire program. 'It took a few years off my life, straightening that one out.'[73]

1960s–present: a model for American healthcare?

The Permanente Group's report of January 1961 was positive, with excess revenue of $450 000. The contingent incentive payment from the Health Plan was averaging $300 000 per quarter, reflecting solid growth. Health Plan membership had increased to 398 000. One third of all eligible federal employees in the northern California region had subscribed to the Plan by the end of 1960. The Medical Group now had its own headquarters at 1924 Broadway in Oakland, formerly the headquarters of Kaiser Industries. By September 1962 Kaiser Permanente had become the single largest private group-practice health plan in the United States, encompassing 12 hospitals and 38 clinics serving 337 000 subscribers (911 000 family members) in California, Oregon and Hawaii. The Kaiser Permanente program was unique in its combination of size and coverage. The closest in size, the Health Insurance Plan of Greater New York, did not provide or pay for hospital care.

By the end of 1965 Kaiser Permanente in northern California had 646 000 enrollees, a net growth of 62% in five years. The 1960s also saw the opening of new regions beyond the Pacific coast and Hawaii. By the 1970s, Kaiser Permanente would be acknowledged as the model for a sea change in healthcare in the USA with the establishment of Health Maintenance Organisations (HMOs). One of the driving forces behind Kaiser Permanente's expansion in the 1960s was the growing participation of employees in capitation prepayment. During the decade the percentage of members for whom the employer paid some or all of the dues increased from 68% to 91%. This underscored an important development in traditional compensation and benefit packages in the United States.

Another driver for expansion was the enrolment in the Health Plan of federal, state and local government employees, stimulated by the Federal Employees Health Benefits Act of 1960, which became the model for similar Californian state legislation. In 1962, the Californian State Employees Retirement Board initiated discussions with Kaiser Permanente and by the end of 1964 a decision was made to begin operations in the State Capital, Sacramento, where Kaiser Foundation Hospitals bought the Arden Hospital. By September 1968 Health Plan enrolment had reached 845 000. The Medical Group had 917 full-time-equivalent physicians, which put the physician–member ratio at 1:921, the most favourable in the history of the program. Including family members, however, would presumably have increased the ratio to around 1:2400.

At the Monterey Conference in 1960, Sidney Garfield had challenged the Medical Group to make three major changes in the conduct of medical care. A new emphasis on maintaining health should be favoured over merely treating sickness. New technology should be used to record and store medical information. And non-physician health personnel should be more integrated into the healthcare process, under physician supervision, in order to extend the physician's effectiveness and efficiency. As will become apparent in this book, these three ideas still exert a strong, formative influence over the Kaiser Permanente healthcare program in Hawaii and in the other regions. In September 1961 a division of Medical Methods Research was established, directed by Morris Collen. Although an internist, Collen had a degree in electrical engineering and a special interest in emerging applications of computer technology to medicine. The division's mandate was, in Collen's words, 'To explore and develop to the fullest extent the "health" aspects of our medical care activities.'[72] The Kaiser Permanente Division of Research, in Oakland, continues that work today.

On 1 January 1969, the board of the Kaiser Permanente Committee elected to proceed with the program's expansion into Denver Colorado and Cleveland Ohio. In March 1971, a three-day Kaiser Permanente Medical Care Program Symposium was held, sponsored jointly by the Association of Medical Colleges, the Commonwealth Fund, and Kaiser Permanente. One month earlier, the Nixon administration proposed legislation to encourage HMOs: 'We suspect,' Clifford Keene told the symposium 'that the similarity of the HMO concept and Kaiser Permanente is more than coincidence. We ourselves don't see Kaiser Permanente as a panacea. We do see it as a valid solution to some long-standing problems. We see it as an evolving method of organising and delivering medical care which is intended to be responsive to the changing needs of the people it serves.'[40]

A year after the proceedings of the symposium were published, over 2.5 million Americans were covered by the Kaiser Permanente program. By 1989, 3000 physicians in the Permanente Medical Group were caring for 2.3 million members in the northern California region in 15 medical centres and 20 satellite offices. New regions had been established in Texas, the middle-Atlantic states, North Carolina, Georgia, the northeastern states and Kansas. Total membership exceeded 6 million.

One of Kaiser Permanente's many contributions to national health policy was its role as a model for the Health Maintenance Organization Act of 1973. 'The law, however, contained provisions unfavourable to the program, especially a too comprehensive benefits package and open enrolment combined with community rating which allowed for adverse selection against the plan, a certain guarantee to make a health plan sick.'[72] Eventually, an alliance of health plans was able to get the act amended and all Kaiser Permanente regions finally became federally qualified HMOs in 1977.

The structure of Kaiser Permanente has not changed fundamentally following the Tahoe Agreement of 1955, though it has continued to evolve. On 2 January 1984 The Permanente Medical Group ceased to be a partnership and became a professional corporation. Among other advantages, incorporation secured physicians' retirement contributions against risk of loss from financial reverses of the program.

Henry J Kaiser died in 1967 at the age of 85. His legacy included some of the largest modern manmade structures on Earth. Sidney Garfield MD died on 29 December 1985, his legacy no less significant to the lives of millions of Americans. 'He captured the principles and significance of prepayment to a group of physicians as a more efficient and effective mechanism for healthcare. He developed the concept against opposition and obstructions that would have been overwhelming to many without his dedication and courage.'[15] The life-works of Kaiser and Garfield had a symbiotic quality. Whereas many of their predecessors, such as the builders of the Central and Union Pacific Railroads, had seen mainly their own narrow financial interests, Kaiser and Garfield understood the close mutual dependency of industry and health and of their respective visions in those fields of endeavour.

Methodology

Qualitative research

To collect data for this study, semi-structured interviews were conducted on Oahu with managers, project team members and front-line clinicians in four teams located in four clinics, and in the Kaiser Permanente hospital. A qualitative approach was taken to this research for four main reasons. First, social studies on medical informatics are comparatively rare, though becoming less so, and there is as yet no consensus concerning the key variables to study, or their relative importance. Second, the opportunity to collect data was delimited by time and resources. We had two weeks in which to conduct interviews and collect any other data. Third, the organisational context was dynamic: we entered the organisation as it was changing from one EMR system to another. Hence a need to be flexible and responsive to opportunities presented in the field. Fourth, the

Table 1.2.   Qualitative and quantitative paradigms

Qualitative	Quantitative
Soft	Hard
Subjective	Objective
Descriptive	Analytical
Inductive	Hypothetico-deductive
Discursive	Numerical
Reflexive	Non-reflexive
Case study	Experimental
Relativistic	Probabilistic
Hermeneutic/interpretive	Logical positivist

Source: adapted from Halfpenny, 1979, and Silverman, 2000[26,71]

intensive character of the study made in-depth ethnographic methods viable and preferable to quantitative data collection and analysis.

Uncertainty concerning the identification of key variables led us to take an exploratory approach to the data collection. We did not expect to produce findings capable of predictive power, although they might reduce the repetition of any errors in the next Kaiser Permanente EMR implementation, which was imminent, but to make a contribution to the growing knowledge of medical informatics implementation challenges and their management. Those unfamiliar with the characteristics of qualitative research will find the table helpful to outline its complementarity with the quantitative paradigm (*see* Table 1.2).

Exploratory research is particularly appropriate when the key variables are unknown or uncertain. In these circumstances a quantitative approach would be unhelpful as the questions asked in a large-scale survey would not be grounded in a valid body of knowledge or robust theoretical frame. The disadvantages of a prematurely designed survey could be severe if respondents completed forced-choice questions that failed to capture the frame of their experience. The results of such a survey might then represent a distorted view of the problem and, if published, prompt further research in a similar vein. Ultimately it is conceivable for a whole problematic to be constructed on the unfounded assumptions of researchers and their customary instruments, bypassing and even corrupting the authentic experience of respondents, and leading to invalid knowledge about the topic. In fact, this tendency can be seen in health informatics research, which is dominated by technical studies that ignore the social dimensions of informatics development and implementation.

In the case of CIS in Hawaii Kaiser Permanente, it was known that the system was to be replaced, but not why. Even when official reasons were disseminated they were couched in diplomatic language and reflected a corporate perspective. It was important to dig into the real reasons why CIS had not been fully implemented in Hawaii, especially as the Colorado region of Kaiser Permanente had been using an earlier version of the CIS system successfully for several years. Had CIS failed to deliver the expected benefits in Hawaii? For what reasons? Were there technical problems in the new version that were not in the Colorado version? Was the apparent failure due to resistance by the clinicians, or other localised causes? How did users in Hawaii assess CIS? And what had they learned from the implementation? It was important to ask these questions in order to learn something from what appeared, superficially at least, to be a very expensive failure, not least as an even bigger investment had been made to adopt a different EMR system. Diagnosing the implementation problems with CIS might help to predict and manage similar difficulties with EpicCare.

Validity and reliability

Validity is a measure of truth or accuracy, the road to which has many pitfalls. Sometimes we doubt the validity of a certain method or instrument to measure what it claims. For instance, does an IQ test really measure intelligence, or only measure our definition of intelligence? We might doubt whether an investigator's interpretations are valid if we suspect that they are supported by inadequate data or that no attempt is made to deal with contrary cases ('anecdotalism'). Unfortunately, field notes or transcripts generated in qualitative research are not usually available to readers to allow them to form their own interpretation of the data, or to set extracts into their original context.[10] An investigator's immersion in the field or data can alter his perception such that he or she may become possessive and resistant to other possible interpretations. 'Or sometimes, the demand by journal editors for shorter and shorter articles simply means that the researcher is reluctantly led only to use "telling" examples.'[71] In the latter regard, we hope that this book adequately compensates for any shortcomings in our original research article published in the *British Medical Journal* and tailored to fit that journal's laconic style.[69]

Reliability 'refers to the degree of consistency with which instances are assigned to the same category by different observers or by the same observer on different occasions'.[27] The issue of consistency arises in qualitative research due to its heavy reliance on the accurate recording, transcription and interpretation of data sources that are inherently ambiguous, in the sense that words and images can be interpreted in diverse ways. It has been argued that once we treat social reality as constantly in flux, i.e. cease to reify what is inherently dynamic, it becomes unnecessary to worry whether our methods of interpretation are reliable.[52] But qualitative research cannot ignore the reliability question. We cannot assume a social world without stable properties. However abstract or elusive, categories such as culture and leadership have consistent, normative effects upon our attitudes, beliefs and behaviour. In terms of its effects, therefore, there does appear to be significant stability in the social world. Indeed, we call that stability *culture*. For reliability to be assessed it is incumbent upon investigators to document their procedures.

We strengthened the reliability of this study in several ways. First, our purposive sample of interviewees was chosen to provide an approximate cross section of occupations and type of involvement in CIS adoption and implementation. All the interviewees were well informed, having specialist knowledge of CIS according to their roles as sponsors, leaders, users and implementation team members. Most had more than one role, balancing their perspectives. In any politically and commercially sensitive research there is a risk of selection bias. Senior leaders in Hawaii Kaiser Permanente invited organisational members to participate in the research. We saw this as necessary to signal internal support for the study and gain access to respondents. As far as we are aware, volunteers were not screened or briefed with a view to influencing sample composition or responses. An absence of selection bias is suggested by the inclusion of individuals with a wide range of views on CIS, from predominantly positive to predominantly negative. Having said that, respondents tended to offer fairly balanced views, which was to be expected from a sample of high average intelligence and educational attainment. Besides, we believe that any unintended selection bias by Hawaii Kaiser Permanente on behalf of the study would tend to have been neutralised by the strongly independent judgement and expression of the respondents: senior physicians (certainly), senior executives (probably, though less so), senior nurses and implementation team members (more circumspectly), respectively.

Second, reliability was strengthened by a systematic approach to the interviews and in two ways. One researcher conducted all the interviews and was therefore able to adopt a *constant comparative method*, meaning that each interview was seen as an opportunity to check and corroborate data collected in previous interviews. The constant comparative approach continued in the data analysis, when any theme arising in interview could be compared and contrasted with themes in the same and other interviews. In addition, the topic guide used in all the interviews lent a general consistency that would have been absent from unstructured conversations. In practice, each interview was a variation on the discursive themes in the topic guide. Within that frame, each interview was approached as a unique event and varied from, in one case, an almost continuous monologue by the respondent requiring minimal intervention by the interviewer to, in other cases, more conventional question and answer based conversations. It is assumed that a certain amount of informal communication between respondents occurred, possibly to debate whether or not the interviewer was an independent researcher as claimed, or an agent of senior management. The frankness exhibited by all respondents suggested that any suspicions any of them might have had were dispelled. On balance the interviewer's Englishness and occupational background, combined with his dual affiliation to Kaiser Permanente's Research Division, on one hand, and UC Berkeley on the other, were probably conducive to candid conversations. This was not by chance: if anyone was vetted for this research it was the interviewer not the interviewed.

Third, all the interviews were transcribed verbatim by the interviewer. This preserved some of the context, atmosphere, tone, mood and other paralinguistic elements of the interviews, helping to inform both transcription and later interpretation. Although this continuity between the stages of the research process is a strength, we recognised a need for external validation of the accuracy and sense of the transcriptions. This task was undertaken by a research assistant familiar with health services research and Hawaii. The RA listened critically to all the original recordings and read the transcripts. Agreement of 100% between the RA and interviewer was reached with minimal changes, indicating that the original transcripts were very accurate. The interview transcripts were also read by all members of the research team who met frequently to discuss their interpretation, which helped to inform the writing of the original book manuscript, and the editing of the final version.

Method

Semi-structured audio-recorded interviews[37,83] were held with a sample of 26 senior clinicians, managers and EMR project team members in Hawaii. An interview prompt sheet was used to standardise the topics covered in the interviews, which lasted from 60 to 90 minutes. The questions sought information about respondents' experiences, opinions and reflections with respect to the planning, implementation and use of the EMR in clinical practice. The topic guide contained a sequence of open questions relating to organisational factors potentially relevant to EMR implementation and care redesign, including organisational culture, leadership, functionality and use, previous IT implementations and effects on processes of care (*see* Appendix A). These questions were formulated in the light of previous qualitative and quantitative studies of organisational readiness to change, organisational culture types and the extent of quality improvement implementation. However, the interview also allowed a free exchange of ideas and experiences of the EMR by respondents. The project was approved by the Kaiser Permanente Hawaii Region Internal Review Board.

The interviews were recorded using digital audio recording equipment. As mentioned above, the recordings were transcribed verbatim. A research assistant independently assessed the accuracy of the transcripts against the recordings. Additional information was obtained by email. As the findings were analysed thematically and inductively[42] they are not presented using a framework derived strictly from the interview questions. Being exploratory, the interviews aimed to discover the most relevant questions to ask about EMR implementation, from the perspective of clinicians and others.

The findings in Chapter 2 are presented largely in respondents' own words by liberal used of verbatim extracts from the interviews. Their spoken language is of course full of grammatical and syntactical irregularities. We prefer the immediacy of actual discourse to correcting 'errors' and removing slang, which are part and parcel of everyday interaction.

The experience of implementation

Introduction

The study findings are organised around three questions:

1 How successful was the implementation?
2 How did participants account for the successes and failures?
3 What were the organisational factors that helped or hindered the implementation?

This chapter presents respondent perceptions of the CIS implementation process, including the perceived failings and successes, reported levels of CIS use, organisational changes resulting from CIS use, and organisational changes resulting from the implementation experience. As will become clear, the software itself was only one focus of the interviews. Respondents commented on different stages of adoption and implementation according to their scope of role and interest, which highlights how perceptions of this complex organisational change often varied across perspectives. We deliberately sought interviews with both primary care clinicians (analogous to general practitioners in the NHS) and specialists; implementation team members; and organisational leaders (analogous to NHS managers). As previously mentioned, we have made a deliberate decision to let respondents speak for themselves as far as possible in this account. Ideally, we would like to have made the full interview transcripts available for interpretation by readers and other researchers. As anonymity was a condition of the study, that was not possible. We have therefore concentrated on composing a narrative that reverses the standard convention of using brief excerpts to illustrate points made by researchers. Instead, after the model of a good qualitative research interview, we intrude into the narrative as little as possible and use multiple extracts to illustrate each theme. The idea behind this style of presentation is to present different perspectives and nuances on the same themes, thus illustrating the heterogeneity of views offered by respondents. It also helps to avoid over-coding. We do not wish to subordinate the interviewees to our own narrative. A large part of our work was to set up procedures and processes to generate the speech that we recorded. The task of coding that speech into themes and selecting excerpts already represents, in our view, a sufficient processing of the 'raw' data generated through the interviews. Clearly any summarising of data entails losses as well as gains. Gained is concision; lost are context and nuance. The reader may judge whether we have struck the right compromise.

Summary of implementation

Implementation of the electronic medical record (CIS) in Hawaii Kaiser Permanente commenced in October 2001, though preparations began some two years earlier. By April 2003, one third of clinics and specialties were fully implemented, the remaining two thirds had read-only access, many also with order entry functionality (termed 'read-only plus'). After two years, a decision was made at group headquarters on the US mainland to halt the implementation and adopt an alternative system starting late 2003. Previously, Kaiser had implemented this CIS successfully in another region and invested considerable effort in planning for the Hawaii CIS implementation. Despite this extensive experience and planning, the Hawaii respondents described a challenging implementation process, variable levels of CIS use, and considerable difficulties adapting to a post-CIS work environment. Overall the implementation process provides several lessons from both perceived successes and failures, which are valuable for any organisation embarking on an IT implementation.

The implementation process: CIS development

Delayed implementation start date

CIS delivery was delayed by 14 months as its conversion from OS2 to Windows NT took much longer (and cost correspondingly more) than anticipated. This delay had important consequences for the vendor–provider relationship, perceptions of Kaiser Permanente leadership, and the CIS users. The delay also prompted physicians to question their own involvement in the software design process and to reaffirm their primary clinical role, as one regional administrator remarked:

> We had a 12-month preparation period, we met monthly, some areas weekly, as we prepared. The product wasn't delivered for another 14 months after we prepared for a year. That affects your culture. This was our national relationship with IBM [system vendor] and expectations that were not met, and a failure on our part to be leaders at the level of working with software developers. Our core skill set is in delivering healthcare, not helping IBM write software.

As preparation and training at the first implementation site were frustrated by the delay in delivering the software, a contingency plan was devised to maintain the program's momentum. Consequently the first site received considerably more preparation for CIS than did subsequent sites, perhaps accounting for different assessments of the application.

During the extended waiting period, the staffing situation at the first site changed significantly, which affected its receptiveness to CIS, as one physician explained:

> The delay had multiple consequences to our whole experience with this. So when we gave the OK to be the first clinic, we had this high achieving team, the all-star cast. A lot of time goes by; lot of things happen in people's lives. And our internist, who was one of the most highly respected internists in the group, needed to go do

some other things. So we were looking at a time when one of our strongest assets was going someplace else. And our paediatrician – the most highly rated as far as patient satisfaction is concerned – also needed to move to neonatology. So the implementation date is shifting and so are the players.

But though morale and performance declined during the delay at the first site, the will to implement remained. Its rationale altered from being the ideal test site, to seeing CIS implementation as a morale boosting exercise:

So when it came time for us to actually start doing CIS, we were at one of our lowest points as far as staff morale and confidence in the quality of care that we were giving. And that turned out to be a blessing, because it gave us something to focus on, a rallying point. This 'Hey, we have a reputation to uphold. We're going to do what it takes to come together and we're going to succeed.' So it helped turn some things around and that was a blessing in disguise.

Product design issues

Respondents reported several concerns with the CIS product design. These concerns included perceived deficiencies in the CIS software, as well as both organisational and technical difficulties in changing the software to fix the identified deficiencies.

Early CIS users in Hawaii found it to be disappointingly slow and inconvenient to use, as one specialty Chief noted:

It definitely did not provide any greater efficiency as far as I'm concerned, and as far as anybody's concerned. Everybody's slower on it; it helps you maybe keep track of your patients a little bit better, but we are definitely not more efficient: we are much, much slower.

One member of the CIS implementation team described it as:

Basically a beta test of something and it was very rocky.

But few respondents condemned the system as a complete failure. Another clinic Chief summarised the ambivalence that most respondents felt towards it – until they learned about its replacement system, EpicCare, when their negative evaluation of CIS hardened:

We knew CIS was coming, so we knew we had to do something. And we knew it was going to be a huge change. It wasn't as bad as I...Alright, it was as bad as I thought it was gonna be. Parts of it weren't as bad, other parts have been worse.

I knew that eventually it would be good, it was just a little bit hard. And now it's really hard because I've seen EpicCare and I think that it is so much better than CIS. But the longer we've been on it [CIS] the easier it is. It's definitely a lot easier now than it was three months ago.

Another Chief commented in more detail on the deficiencies of CIS:

Within a few weeks it was very apparent that this product was not what one would expect of a state-of-the-art system. It turned out to be a glorified word processor, with a useful way to order medications and do orders. But the main thing physicians do is document their notes, and it wasn't a very good word processor. It didn't have some of the most basic things that you would expect from the word processor you would use at home. Things like macros for repetitive tasks, which can save you a lot of time. The way that the note was formatted, spell checking were not included. It wasn't giving me any information that I didn't have before – maybe I had to toggle between the lab system and the diagnostic imaging system; but that wasn't that difficult – it was all on the mainframe. So one of the other failures or mistakes that I saw was that the people who were implementing CIS couldn't give a convincing argument as to how it would really benefit the end user.

A specialty Chief also criticised the utility of CIS for clinical note-taking:

The one major thing that we really wanted was the ability to take a previous note, bring the data forward, and create a new note based on the old data. Most systems allow you to say, 'Here is last week's note: it's now today's note. Make any changes you want or not and say it's today's note.' So if it took you an extra 15 minutes on the first visit to take the history, but it saves you 5 minutes in each subsequent visit then…But if you have to reinvent the wheel at every visit you lose a lot of the benefit.

Important discrepancies were also found between the software expected and specified by clinicians and the software actually delivered, as a senior administrator noted:

And then there were changes in the product that was delivered that were very unexpected: think 'Non-starts'. It's like, 'You said you were gonna deliver X, you delivered Y, Y can't be worked with. You must go back and redo this to deliver X.'

More discouraging still was the realisation that many desired changes were prohibitively slow and costly to achieve. This information quickly spread through the region, severely damaging confidence in the system. A member of the implementation team noted how this put regional leaders in a more difficult position:

It was pretty clear that this product had a lot of problems – from our very first site. Technically it went up fine. There were a bunch of software problems. But the tool itself was not as good as people expected to see. And in an organisation, that spreads like wildfire. So it was very difficult for the leadership to stand up in front of everybody and say: 'We are going in this direction; this is the right way to go', when very credible people – we picked very credible people to do the initial install – were saying, 'You know, we can do this but if this is all there is we are in big trouble.'

An implementation team member observed, bluntly:

Overlaying all this was the fact that this application's a turkey. So that's superimposed on all the problems you'd have with trying to implement this kind of change, even with a good product.

Some physicians felt that the added value of CIS over older and still operational systems did not justify its adoption. Consequently, one specialty Chief reported very low CIS utilisation in his specialty:

Do they all use CIS? A better question is: Do any of them? Everybody's been trained on it. I've never actually seen a nurse open it up. I've seen the physicians open it up rarely, when they don't have any other choice; when they turned off printed and said you have to go to CIS to find the chart notes. – Because everything else is available on the mainframe, which everyone has been using since before CIS came here. The mainframe gives you lab, radiology reports, dictations, demographics; those are the major functions. We then have a PACS [picture archiving and communication system] for looking at certain X rays. The only thing that CIS added was if a physician generated a note in CIS, once they turned off the printing that was the only place it was available.

That some physicians resorted to CIS only when they had no other choice might suggest that previous systems should have been withdrawn from service. But that might not have been practicable during the rollout, when clinics and specialties using CIS would still need access to data on old systems, and to communicate with other sites awaiting implementation.

Another respondent was disappointed by his inability to use CIS as a research database to evaluate care:

'From what I heard, this was the whole reason for the project. We were going to get all this data that we could make healthcare decisions on.'

He also commented on the 'workarounds' users devised to circumvent some of CIS's problems:

Even when people got better at using CIS, they gave up a lot of its benefits. They used transcription, or copy and paste, or used some workaround: anything they could do to get the day done.

These concerns with the software are likely to be present in all implementations, for there will never be a perfect software package or information system for all users, in all situations. Indeed, how organisations identify and respond to the perceived CIS deficiencies is instructive.

This raises two issues of systems design: first, that ingenious users will tend to find ways to short circuit the inconvenient features of any system, and second, that system designers tend not to learn from such ingenuity, as neither side communicates with the other effectively. Users will always circumvent formal systems or functions that work against their interests.

CIS development: getting changes made in the CIS software

Respondents noted that fixing these perceived deficiencies required an inordinate length of time, and fabulous expense. The difficulty in systematically identifying and fixing the shortcomings did not endear CIS to its users:

And the changes to the system were really slow. That was something we weren't prepared for. It was months and months and months before things that were wrong with the system could be reprogrammed.

Not surprisingly, respondents reported that the lack of an efficient process for fixing problems frustrated clinicians. The implementation team initially became a target for some of the criticism of CIS. Team members deflected some of that criticism towards Kaiser Permanente national leadership who had authorised the adoption decision. The vendor also received criticism for its perceived failure to respond to the problems identified by local users.

> *The criticism that people were making of CIS was very well placed. I tried to turn it by telling people, 'Don't rail against it: your real question is to ask the people that make these decisions, "Can you get it changed? Over what timeframe? Will I be involved? Will you get user input?"' Unfortunately, the national organisation wasn't able to respond to that at all.*

While there was a process for identifying CIS problems, there was no consensus on how to address these problems. As the number of CIS problems increased, differences in organisational priorities appeared to make addressing user problems more difficult. Initially, there were weekly debriefings with clinicians to discuss any CIS problems. These were then translated into recommendations for improvement at monthly meetings with Kaiser Permanente HQ in Oakland California. But respondents reported feeling that feedback was quickly discarded. This annoyed the regional administrators, clinicians and implementation team in Hawaii, and eroded their faith in the national organisation. In the words of one regional administrator:

> *We were promised that our weekly debriefs with physicians and nurses who were using the system would be translated into clinical recommendations. We flew people to California monthly to deliver those recommendations for a period of 12 months. It's very disheartening for the national leadership to say, 'Oh. Here's 12 months of clinical input that actually we're going to make of secondary importance for now, because we're looking at our return on investment.' I'm just saying that before we had new national leadership, we weren't being listened to in the same way.*

A member of the implementation team explained how that apparent reversal in priorities created frustration in Hawaii, and exacerbated the problem of trying to promote a 'clunky' application:

> *We and representatives from all the other regions who were going to be using CIS spent hours in meetings, talking about enhancements: which were the best ones; which were the [ones] users [were] asking for. Each one had several pages explaining how it would work and we prioritised those, we argued about them, we put them on different lists. All that work basically got scrapped. Executive decisions were made to limit the scope to things that would increase revenue, that would do a better job of coding, and that would make the system scaleable to be used in places like California – all of which are extremely important organisational imperatives, but along the way the usability and the user input literally got X'd off the page. And that was a very, very difficult thing to deal with because we had been telling people from the beginning, 'We know it's not perfect, but give us your ideas: we will help to make it better.' And that clearly changed about a year and a half ago, when we were told that all the work of the scope committee was no longer in scope.*

One Chief observed:

> *As we made suggestions to improve things they were just ignored and their time schedule went on its merry way.*

Another Chief noted:

> *It's been a growing dissatisfaction and irritation as requests for functional*

> *improvements get either rejected outright or pushed back to future releases, and that general feeling of 'No one is listening to us'. We were kind of the alpha-site. When you're an alpha-site they are supposed to listen to you. I mean you take on the challenge of using a piece of software that is very new, you expect bugs, you expect problems; but you also expect to be listened to and say: 'OK, this isn't working: let's go and fix this' and I think the general feeling is that they didn't listen.*

Why did respondents feel that headquarters stopped listening to delegates from Hawaii? Perhaps the two sides operated under different paradigms and priorities. Consequently, they did not share a common understanding of the situation and failed to communicate effectively. Asked about relations between Hawaii Kaiser Permanente and Kaiser Permanente HQ, a senior member of the implementation team replied:

> *I think the problems that we had with the national organisation – and it may not be their fault because they were constrained – their priorities were to get something rolled out under a certain budget, in a relatively short timeframe. They had difficulty dealing with being told, 'Hey look, you gotta fix this because it really makes it hard for users'. And because of those constraints they really weren't set up to deal with that. And to an extent they didn't understand it. And to some extent their hands – the people making the decisions – were tied by people above them that were driving money, you know, very high in the organisation, that were focused on budget.*

This situation may have also have hindered the effective communication of Hawaiian clinical concerns and priorities to the system vendor, IBM. The same respondent went on to address the Kaiser Permanente–IBM relationship:

> *I think the problems that the national organisation had with the vendor were to do with the [pause] I think they underestimated the ability of the vendor to solve technical problems. I think national tried to do too much on their own. And I think they made a fundamental mistake in selecting a vendor that really didn't have a market, and wasn't putting any R&D money into improving the products. So you can see the difference, where you have a market-driven vendor [Epic] that's putting a lot of their money into R&D; and IBM – any improvements we had to pay for. So we're paying for their entire development [costs]. And that was a fundamental mistake: I think the highest levels of the organisation made a mistake in the selection process. In my opinion I don't think they [acted with] due diligence. They simply made incorrect assessments.*

Differences in priorities also will exist in all large organisations and during all large scale IT implementations. In a baseline study of four hospital Trusts in England, in the context of the UK NHS National Programme for Information Technology (NPfIT), Hendy *et al.*[28] noted five main factors affecting the implementation of NPfIT:

- *Communication problems:* Implementation sites suffered problems of poor communication and coordination. This exacerbated the implementation challenges for NPfIT. Moreover, respondents reported poor communication between NPfIT programme office and implementation sites, and local advice being ignored.
- *Financial effects – opportunity costs:* Many Trusts experienced severe financial difficulties. Understandably, therefore, some cash-strapped Trusts delayed

implementation in favour of more immediate priorities, and pending decisions about additional central funding.

- *Performance ratings:* The opportunity costs of implementation were further exacerbated where a Trust had a low performance rating (0 or 1 star) under the (discredited) star-rating system. Should such a Trust invest in its future performance ratings, or NPfIT – which would further reduce its productivity, at least in the short/medium term?
- *Legacy systems:* The NPfIT reversed the previous policy of local IT procurement, which produced a proliferation of IT architecture. NPfIT implementation threatened losses in functionality during the transition between old and new systems. They were also cautious about ending contracts with existing suppliers. As previous NHS policies, such as competitive tendering, had shown, contractors often prefer to stick with existing suppliers than switch for what might be only short-term gains at best. Moreover, the hidden costs incurred in switching suppliers are insufficiently acknowledged by a free market model.
- *Timetable for implementation:* The Care Records software would require most Trusts to replace their existing patient administration systems. In London this was projected to take up to 5 years.

Hendy *et al.* conclude, albeit on the basis of scant preliminary evidence, that each NHS implementation site varied in its circumstances and implementation challenges; the process of implementation of the NPfIT was suboptimal, and the timetable unrealistic. At time of writing, 23 leading computer science academics have written to the Health Select Committee, highlighting their concerns about NPfIT and calling for an independent assessment of its basic technical viability. Meanwhile, a BBC *File on 4* survey found that 85% of doctors agreed with them. Only 4% disagreed.

We did not interview any of the national organisation or CIS implementation leaders, thus this report is inherently one-sided. Nevertheless, the perceptions of our respondents are instructive; these perceptions drove subsequent attitudes and responses to the CIS implementation.

For example, some clinicians had tolerant attitudes towards the initial deficiencies of the CIS – attitudes which stiffened markedly when they learned of obstacles preventing their correction. One Chief explained:

> *The system was too rigid and clunky. What made us devalue the system was not that it happened, but that they couldn't fix it. It seemed like with CIS, if you wanted to make a change, it would take six months and cost anywhere from two to ten million dollars.*

Another physician was frustrated by a lack of responsiveness to opportunities to enhance CIS and thereby improve care processes:

> *I mean we were just ready: we could just see the power behind it. But the one area that we still think that there's tremendous power, and nothing has been done, is the prenatal record. We actually thought we could automate our prenatal records, so we could dump all the paper. We still have that issue up in L&D [Labour and Delivery]. Here that's not a problem. But every other clinic, if the patient got seen today and then goes to L&D tonight, that note is not around for us to see. And we wanted to fix that and it could be, it just cost too much money to work on and finally get a prenatal record that works. It's so standard, so standard: it's sad that*

we can't do it. I don't get why it can't be done but they quoted two million dollars. It was like, 'Never mind'.

Care delivery issues: nothing and everything to do with CIS

Implementing CIS reverberated throughout Hawaii Kaiser Permanente, affecting care delivery issues in numerous ways that were not, and to some degree could not have been, anticipated. In this manner, CIS implementation became a lens passed meticulously over the organisation, revealing a hitherto limited knowledge of existing care delivery processes and workflows. Here, we describe some examples of care delivery challenges identified during the implementation process.

The implementation program reverberated throughout the organisation by uncovering a host of operational issues. This ripple effect gave rise to a truism: *It has nothing to do with CIS, and everything to do with CIS.* The unanticipated effects of the implementation were likened to opening Pandora's Box.* According to mythology, Mercury left a certain box in Pandora's safekeeping, which he warned her never to open. Eventually, overcome with curiosity, Pandora opened the box and out flew all the evils of the world. But the last thing to escape from the box was Hope. So what were the hidden problems released by CIS and was there any redeeming factor there too?

An implementation team member noted that CIS implementation magnified anomalies and inefficiencies:

> *There was a lot of stuff that came up that had nothing to do with CIS but had everything to do with CIS. Nothing to do with CIS software, but a lot of the operational stuff that came to the surface because of CIS that we had to manage.*

Several respondents noted this disclosive function of CIS. The preparatory work, the process of implementing the application, and its later consequences all cast a new and critical light on activities that had previously been concerns of individual physicians, but now took on a systemic, regional significance. According to one implementation team member:

> *Implementing CIS really did open up Pandora's Box. It caused us to look at every single workflow process within clinic operations, because it touches almost everything. And then it fed into the billing. Now it's starting to touch on all the backend processes as well. CIS tends to bring your hidden problems to the fore. Things that were there before, but now, after 20 years, it's critical that we solve because it has implications for our deployment.*

Another implementation team member noted a similar effect:

> *Many of the things that have changed and been learned have nothing to do with CIS and yet everything to do with CIS, because it opened Pandora's Box.*

---

*We own that it was the interviewer who introduced Pandora's Box. One might object that this led these respondents. But leading is part of any interview. Unless the interviewer remains silent – and even then the setting provides cues, this effect is inevitable and necessary.

The Pandora's Box effect was part of the complex challenge to prepare clinics to transfer to the electronic world by studying their workflows, as recalled by another member of the implementation team:

> One of the things we did in order to roll out CIS is you have to really study the workflow. So we had gained a lot in the efficiencies in workflow, and the agreements that physicians needed to express to each other about how they do their work, how the handoffs work. So that we made tremendous improvements because those things that had never been expressed before, like, 'So, how am I going to get this to you?' And, 'How are we going to work together on this?' happened.
>
> The other thing about any automated system is it magnifies your inefficiencies and you have to address it because you have to have new processes.

This close analysis of errors brought with it a corresponding escalation of work to implement CIS, as another member of the team related from personal experience:

> I knew it was going to be hard work, but it's turned out to be much more detail-oriented, and a lot more work than I anticipated because of things that weren't working right. Such a lot of work just to get one line item on that list checked off. The list was formidable in the beginning and as you learned more about what those items meant, then you realised 'Oh my God: that's a lot of work.'

Neither health providers nor the CIS team could ignore the issues thus raised.
  If CIS magnified discrepancies and the workload of implementation, it also intensified problems elsewhere in the system, as one respondent noted:

> I think the other lesson learned is that – and we've seen this so often – CIS is going to magnify any challenges you have that are non-CIS related. It's a huge magnifier. If you have access issues, we're going to magnify that when we come in and reduce your schedule. And you need to build in some fat to deal with that.

A more optimistic view is that standardising practices could help lead to qualitative improvements in processes, by disclosing unnecessary variation in practices and agreeing to adopt the most efficient procedures, as one Chief reported:

> I think when we all got together it actually showed people how differently they practised. I think we all kind of thought that we were all the same – and maybe your style's a little bit different from mine, but when we actually looked at it, you know, just to have an I&D [Incision and Drainage], there were seven different ways that the MAs [medical assisstants] had to set up an I&D kit, because we all wanted our own different thing.

Identity and access

To get users onto the application in a timely way was a key challenge. A subgroup formed to work on computer access for new hires, for which certificates had to be issued from national office. This certification gave rise to basic issues about user names. If someone's email name did not match their legal name, a user certificate could not be issued, as one implementation team member commented:

There's a question about what is a legal name? Is it the name on your medical license, or is it the name on your driver's license? Because when you sign a chart in paper nobody cares. You scribble something, who cares, right? But in the electronic world it spells it out, and then all of a sudden, if I never changed my license and my license is under my maiden name, the lawyers are coming up and saying, 'You have to sign a legal record with the name on your license!' So we are in these huge battles about what is the name that should be on our records. That flows across Social Security and everything, because you can't have people using five different names.

This deceptively simple issue caused many delays to implementation because the ambiguity over a single user name halted implementation at the entire site. As some Chiefs were reluctant to apply pressure on individuals to update their licenses, these delays could be protracted.

Scope of practice

A person's electronic identity and associated security profile (which gave access to CIS), and the name on their medical license related to the kinds of clinical tasks they could legally undertake, their scope of practice, as a member of the implementation team noted:

The functionality of CIS was dependent upon an individual's security profile for access to the system. Well, that needed to be correlated to the person's scope of practice. We never had a formal infrastructure for the nursing supervisors to manage that. Now we had to because they didn't have access to CIS, or to the places that they needed to be in CIS, if we weren't clear what their scope was. So we had to introduce and manage scope of practice, and help them to redesign the workflow.

The processes of preparation for CIS implementation revealed that many nurses and medical assistants had been routinely conducting procedures that might have been questionable in the context of their scope of practice as defined by State law. This problem was partly attributable to a drift in job roles at clinic level, but also due partly to the development of an earlier version of CIS in the Colorado region, as another implementation team member noted:

That caused problems with CIS because it was so specific to the Colorado region. It was designed off of the scope of practice laws in Colorado. Some of the functions and features were hard to implement in Hawaii because the scope of practice laws are different. And we would have encountered those issues in the other regions as well.

For example, a nurse might routinely order urine analyses for patients with probable urinary tract infections, without seeking a doctor's order; or alter a patient's drug dosage. Or a medical assistant might conduct a simple diagnostic test, as a senior administrator described:

Scope of practice for a medical assistant or a registered nurse may be different across states. For example, can an MA [medical assistant] adequately perform a monofilament sensate testing of a diabetic's foot? Well the answer is yes, absolutely, they can do a great job. Is it in their scope of practice as it relates to state law? Not at all – only a registered nurse is allowed to do that type of diagnostic testing.

Although benign and helpful to the workflow, therefore, some such practices were seen to increase the organisation's vulnerability to possible litigation, or investigation by State and Federal authorities, as an implementation team member described:

> My view of that is very much coloured by my past experience. When I was working for [one of Hawaii Kaiser Permanente's competitors], the FBI came in and seized files. Medicare fraud was the charge and you are talking about a meticulous audit of records and charges, and so I think the risk is very real. And the threat is that we are now going into HIPAA* compliance. And as an organisation we have to decide what risk we are going to assume. I think that in this age of whistle-blowers, you have to run a pretty tight ship.

This was a view reiterated by another implementation team member:

> Because of the risk of litigation we have to keep to a higher standard. If you don't have those systems and don't enforce them, then you are in big trouble. You can't cover anything up in the electronic environment: it's there for everybody to see, so it puts a microscope on everything that you do, and it holds you to that higher standard.

The extent of the problem varied between locations, as one implementation team member remarked:

> You kind of don't know what you don't know until you go into a clinic. I can think of particular clinics we went into and the scope of practice specialists were just like, 'OK, I was there five minutes, I found 20 violations and I just decided to focus on the top three!' You know, I don't panic and run screaming from the room: this is the reality of business.

This finding poses a question about the extent of scope of practice violations in the wider healthcare sector, both in the US and in other countries. At least one implementation team member thought the problem was widespread:

> The process of analysing the workflow, as preparation for CIS, began to show up local practices, nurses doing what could be interpreted as medical practice. I think that's common outside our organisation.

Questionable scopes of practice could not be translated into computerised procedures. Thus it became necessary to retrain staff, some of which might have been exceeding their licenses for a long time. This threatened the morale of some providers who had appreciated learning new techniques and extending their skills, usually with the encouragement of doctors, only to be told that they could not continue to practise those skills.

Hence the detailed analysis and documentation of actions required to prepare for CIS had focused attention on who, precisely, does what. The issue generated anxiety particularly among some of the nursing staff, who even feared to lose their licenses, as an implementation team member observed:

---

*The (US) Health Insurance Portability and Accountability Act (HIPAA), passed in 1996, intended to ensure appropriate protection of confidential healthcare information. Wide-ranging in scope, covering both storage and transmission of this data, as well as stipulating comprehensive compliance requirements, HIPAA is having a substantial impact upon the healthcare sector.

It was very threatening to the nurses, especially to the RNs, because they felt suddenly like they were being exposed. Like they had been sometimes doing things all along that we had said it was OK for them to, but it really wasn't and so there was a lot of talk about their licenses at risk. There was a lot of this drama around it. We had to do a lot of counselling-down and saying, 'Listen, the reason we are doing this is so everybody will be safer.'

In most of these cases, nurses were following formal or informal protocols which, for the sake of expediency, sanctioned a step or more beyond their scope of practice. This raises the familiar dichotomy between the formal and informal aspects of organisation.[63] The formal organisation relates to how things are laid down in official documents, manuals, organisation charts and so forth, whilst the informal organisation relates to how people actually interact and do their work, often ignoring formal boundaries. Both organisational modes are necessary. Without the informal organisation the formal organisation could not function. The informal organisation compensates for actions that are not specified by the formal organisation but are still needed for operational and social reasons. In other words, the formal organisation is virtual, the informal organisation is its actuality.

A case in point would be the patient calling in with urinary tract infection symptoms, as one Chief noted:

Well technically, the advice nurse taking that information should not order a UA [urine analysis] because she hasn't had a formal doctor's order. However, in point of fact that really is what we want. So in this new computerised system, where everything is carefully documented, in terms of the time of when things were ordered, who then countersigns it, etc., etc., we had to create some workarounds. We got around it by creating protocols. We created a UTI [urinary tract infection] protocol for example: that, with these certain symptoms, the nurse was authorised to do certain things and then we could sign off on it. We've done the same thing with results management. We created a protocol for nurses to review results and within what parameters.

In this case, implementing CIS meant adjusting the boundaries of formal and informal practice, formalising some hitherto informal aspects of care to bring them more clearly within the scope of state law.

Loss of flexibility

However, some clinicians felt that CIS demanded excessive formalisation of roles and responsibilities. One Chief complained that the increased visibility and accountability imposed by CIS had turned physicians into very expensive clerks:

Another thing that bothers me – and it bothers a lot of people who are not into CIS – is the amount of work the doctor has to do. And basically what CIS has done, in its rigidity, has made the most expensive employee a clerk, in terms of input of data, or input of order, or input of notes.

I never understood why people can't just input stuff into the note, even diagnoses, and the doctor who looks at it at the end of the day can sign that note, and by signing it verifies that he or she agrees with everything above. But right now, we have to input all of everything, even orders. And I can understand some of the orders, like the narcotics. But I got a nurse who says: 'You have to input the order', whereas in the past I would say: 'Listen, why don't you call in some Vicodin 'cause they're hurting?' So she would say: 'OK.' So she would call it in. Now, I have to say, 'No, you can't call it in.' I have to open up CIS; call up this patient's chart; input that medication; click send, submit, whatever; sign it…Those are inefficiencies that don't make sense to me.

So the verbal order part of it has kind of disappeared. If they were to mimic the processes and efficiencies within the way we do things, sure I can see how the lawyers would never let us do certain things, but I'd be willing to input the narcotics if they'd allow everything else to be put through, without me doing it all myself.

These 'inefficiencies' could be interpreted as part of a wider administrative trans-formation of medicine from a verbal to a recorded practice. Or, more precisely, to see CIS as a novel infrastructure designed to exert greater organisational control by a more accurate classification of diseases, on the one hand, and their appro-priate courses of treatment on the other. In that respect CIS would have been recognised by Michel Foucault[22] as just another disciplinary technology involved in transforming society from domination by traditional modes of power to a more rational distribution of life in modernity, including medicine. But such a controlling infrastructure tends to contradict the notion of clinical autonomy – itself at once a generic professional demand and a rearguard action against the gradual erosion of traditional professional privileges – to which the verbal order bears witness. The verbal order is a demonstration of power in all three senses identified classically by Lukes:[6,50]

1 exercised publicly to secure a decision in situations where there is observable conflict
2 exercised privately to determine what shall be open to dispute and
3 internalised, institutional norms concerning what is disputable and indis-putable.

The verbal order combines all three aspects: doctor simultaneously demands an action, makes it clear that s/he does not seek to debate any scope of practice implications raised, and reinforces institutional norms concerning whose pre-rogative and responsibility it is to make these medico/administrative decisions. Physicians used to issuing verbal instructions no doubt value their flexibility but are less accountable for their actions than those who issue a written order.

One implementation team member reported tensions over scope of practice issues between physician and nurse leads. This tension was resolved by formalising certain desired local practices under protocols as previously mentioned:

We certainly had tension between the nursing lead for the organisation and the physician lead. Because the physician leads who had very successful medical assist-ants, [and] who were doing some of these things, they wanted to be able to continue because that helped them see more patients. So once we clarified the law, if we wanted to do things by protocol and had a written document then we were in much better stead.

Other respondents supported the clarification of roles and responsibilities that CIS implementation had helped to establish. In one Chief's opinion:

There's not the lack of clarity about what your job description is, and what you should be doing and what the expectation is. Whereas I think before there would be. Sometimes a nurse might feel uncomfortable doing something that may have fallen on the borderline of her scope of practice. Now she has something to back her up.

The electronic In-Basket

The electronic In-Basket function was a common cause of concern among physicians. The results of lab tests ordered by physicians were routed into their electronic In-Baskets, abolishing paper results. The In-Basket required the reader to acknowledge with mouse clicks each result, regardless of whether it was normal or abnormal. But that was not how physicians were accustomed to handling paper results, as one Chief explained:

There are two parts to it. The first is seeing the lab results. And it takes longer to see them with CIS than if you were just leafing through a stack of papers, an abnormal result catching your eye, circle it, then rip that one off and put it in a stack of things that you're going to deal with later. In a matter of seconds you've gone through a fairly large number of labs. Whereas in CIS for each individual result you have to do at least two or three clicks to acknowledge that you have seen it, which is not very time-efficient. There are many lab tests that we do that we're not really interested in the exact result: we're just interested in the general trend, whether it is normal or not normal. And so you could look at a collection of labs on a piece of paper and just say, 'OK, all those liver tests are normal', whereas with CIS I have to click through each individual test to acknowledge that.

Another clinician made a similar complaint:

Internal medicine will literally get 50 sheets of paper – labs, with three or four labs on one sheet. Here's one with four labs: in CIS this one shows up and I've got to click on it five times; then this one will show up and five times. So actually I have 20 keystrokes here, just to get rid of this one page.

   OK, you're gonna to make design errors – but to fix it took forever. Almost as soon as it showed up we knew there was a problem. You know, 'It's gonna take ten million dollars and six months'. They installed the fix two weeks ago. And we identified this last summer.

This again makes the point that it wasn't just the dysfunctional aspects of CIS that undermined confidence, but the inability to correct quickly the problems identified early in the implementation. We do not know exactly why the improvement to the In-Basket took so long. The high cost, however, is more clearly attributable to IBM who, if not just exploiting the situation, must have faced considerable technical challenges to alter the In-Basket function. This may hold an important lesson for other software designers in the healthcare sector.

Heterogeneous responses to the In-Basket

How different clinics, specialties and hospital departments addressed the

In-Basket problem highlights the heterogeneity of Hawaii Kaiser Permanente culture, in terms of practitioner background and ethnicity, clinic size, location and mix of staff, specialties, populations served, capacity, individual personalities, and leadership. This is not to diminish the importance of the commonalities that also define the Hawaii region, in contrast with Kaiser Permanente's mainland regions. The importance of that heterogeneity relates to the different and varyingly successful experiences that each implementation site had with CIS. These distinctive experiences were invoked in many respondent narratives. As one Chief explained, implementation at a large city clinic was very different from that at a small clinic in affluent suburbs:

> [One large city] clinic, which is a group of internists, goes onto CIS and they have all kinds of problems with it. They have never been able to reach 100% of the number of patients that they had prior to CIS. There's this thing called the In-Basket in CIS, where your results show up and you have to deal with them. They've chosen to turn off that function of CIS because they felt that it just took too much time and it didn't really add any value to them. Which is a very different perspective from my perspective. My perspective was that you're turning off one of the few things that makes this thing different from what you had before; one of the few things that possibly could add value to you.

Other clinics and specialties did not turn off the In-Basket function, partly because they may have held different ideas about what constituted good practice and quality improvement, and partly also because they were under different pressures and constraints. Some clinics turned the bottleneck of the In-Basket into an opportunity to reallocate tasks, relieving physicians of its more mechanical demands, as a member of the implementation team described:

> So a lot of groups decided, 'Well actually, I don't need to see normals – except in certain situations. The nurses can get rid of all my normals.' So they set up a results management system that we never did before, where the nurses would actually go in at certain times of day and they would get rid of as many normals as they could out of those In-Baskets. And most of the time the doctors didn't even need to know that.

One Chief explained how this innovation worked in one clinic:

> What we're talking about – the bigger picture – is not about using CIS, that's not our goal. Our goal is to move to an electronic medical record. There are different ways of thinking and interacting. One of the significant changes that occurred in our clinic has been the use of that In-Basket and management of results. It allows us to use an RN as our results manager to screen the labs and do a lot of the legwork involved in following them up. So if I see an abnormal potassium level and I need to follow it up with the patient – and I often play phone tag with the patient – [to] tell them whatever I need to tell them. But now with everything in that In-Basket it's simpler for me to see the abnormal lab and give explicit instructions to my results manager – and it's all documented – and my results manager can do all those things while I am doing other things.
>   So that has changed how we practise and it has helped us to think of ourselves more as a team of physicians who are taking care of a group of patients as opposed to me and my practice, and my colleague with her practice – instead of the four silos.

It's more apparent that we need to interact with each other, and we do because when one of us is away we're covering their In-Basket, and we know each other's patients better and each other's practice styles better. It gives us opportunities to discuss how we practise. So that's one of the cultural changes that have come with use of this electronic medical record.

The task of redesigning lab results management related to other issues, such as state scope of practice and licensing questions. These issues, apparently, needed to be resolved by lawyers at national level, as a member of the implementation team noted:

For example, just sorting the In-Basket: that was a big scope of practice issue: 'Well, why can't an MA go into my electronic In-Basket and preview the stuff and let me know what's a priority to look at for the day and what's not?' Well that was a huge hurdle for us to get over, until finally some savvy lawyer looked at it with the Program Office and said: 'It's just sorting. You're not asking the MA to do any kind of medical assessment, they're just sorting the work.'

One clinic Chief thought the advantages of the In-Basket outweighed the disadvantages:

Like the labs that come in and the X-rays; you don't lose 'em. If you lost a piece of paper, then nobody ever saw it, and nobody ever did anything about it. At least this way you're sure that somebody has seen it and somebody has checked it off and done something about it. And then the medications and the chronic patients: you can sort of keep track of what you're doing with them. It's a little bit better for patient care.

Templates

The template function of CIS was designed to provide physicians with a menu of options for typical health conditions and care plans. The physician would work through a relevant template, selecting appropriate tests, treatments, etc. Having completed the page, the physician would then 'commit' it and all the unselected options fell away leaving behind a care plan for the patient. Different sets of templates were designed for different specialties. Hawaii Kaiser Permanente physicians formed teams charged with specifying the templates they needed; their work was then translated by IBM into the software application. What in theory appeared a logical procedure was in practice not very successful. Some physicians failed to find their design work reflected in the templates delivered by IBM. This may have been an effect of different assumptions and expectations between physicians and programmers; an effect exacerbated by physicians not having a version of CIS software to work on, as one Chief described:

We worked very hard on templates. And we spent hours on these things; put a lot of hard work into them. But that work was not reflected in the templates that we actually received from IBM. We ended up using templates that came from Colorado region, where they were using [an older version of] CIS. We also were hampered by not having the software to look at. So we were thinking, theoretically, 'Well this is how you're going to handle a piece of information that comes to you.' But that's very difficult to do without seeing what happens when you actually click something and what will it actually look like and where do things go. The fact that we didn't get our software until later and later and later, that affected the effectiveness of all this hard work that we were putting in.

The utility of templates was found to vary across specialties, with general surgery and obstetrics and gynaecology (OB/GYN) being more amenable than primary care, internal medicine, or paediatrics. Informants attributed this variation to differences in the types of health problems presented. One subspecialty Chief noted:

When we started the CIS stuff, I thought that specialty care would implement easier, because you have this problem-based style or expectation that lends itself to computerisation. The way we input the data into this thing: you can kind of structure it, because the sets of questions, the sets of data that you require – problem/ solution – are kind of set. And you can standardise them easier. [But] when you do primary care, you click on these issues and by the time you get to the bottom of the barrel, it's hard to figure out what they've done – because they're not really solving a problem.

The algorithmic character of care in surgery and OB/GYN was also contrasted with internal medicine, where, as another physician noted:

You're dealing with multiple, multiple problems, and here you are trying to go through four or five templates and then come out the end – you probably can't figure out where you've been. I think actually for OB/GYN, even as primary care, we usually do one or two problems at a time, we don't do five and ten problem lists that go on from one visit to the next. So when I get four or five problems it gets hard for me to keep using one template and another.

OB/GYN adapted fairly easily to CIS because we started with the top 10 problems that we deal with most often. Then we went to the next 10, and it really wasn't that hard to do.

Whereas general surgery was characterised as a focused discipline, internal medicine was seen as diffuse and irreducible to rational, linear programming. A clinic manager summarised the differences thus:

The tool seemed to be designed that you came in for a focused visit. Well in internal medicine that's not their usual visit. I don't know whether to stop in the middle of the template and address your concern about your back problems, or if I can just say: 'Hold it there a minute, I need to get to the end of my template, because it doesn't allow me to...' So I think the design of the system didn't really support the internal medicine physician.

Other clinic managers and implementation team members confirmed this assessment and also emphasised the importance of assessing the receptiveness of a clinic or discipline:

Now, we needed to get a speciality care up. 'OK, we're having some problems with primary care: what happens when you do a specialty department?' Well, General Surgery was willing to go up and go full functionality and actually it went very, very smoothly. So I did approach it differently. I had to look for those people who were at a state of readiness and willingness.

It works very well for a specialised department where you've got standard templates and standard things that you're looking at, whereas with primary care, it's the whole waterfront.

It was suggested that, if they designed the templates around the ideal visit learned in medical school, rather than the exigencies and inevitable compromises of actual medical practice, then internal medicine's problems with templates may have been partly of their own making.

OB/GYN would say: 'We're very simple people. We like things very simple.' So that was how they designed their templates. Internal medicine went for the ideal model. If you came in for the ideal visit, and we should do this and this and this and this and this, and so these templates were like...You might have done that when you were a resident, or a medical student, but you had an hour for your visit and you were expected to cover all this. The current internal medicine physician has 15 minutes and is supposed to get to the main point. And the way the system supported it, it required them to get to their answer and then collect supporting data, which doesn't work. I mean it doesn't work in any kind of science.

One specialty Chief was critical of the template function for failing to provide a way of editing previous templates:

One of the things the system does is create a template, where you can make some selections: 'How many times do you xxxxx in the day?' – check a box, etc. All these questions can be clicked through. My suggestion was that once completed, let me save that template in a free state, resurrect it any time I want, make a few changes, and then commit it. Once you commit the completed template, everything that you checked off becomes part of the note and everything else drops away. We wanted to save the pre-committed template so that we could go back to it and update it. It doesn't seem that difficult to do, but it wasn't a priority because it didn't solve the corporate issues – from what I understand.

Either one could work. You could type a note and just copy and paste it, in which case you lose the coded data but you retain the text. Or within a template you retain the coded data, then that becomes very easy to go back and mine later on, but also you can resurrect it, make whatever changes you want, based on whatever you have done and their responses to the treatment.

The template function appeared to have incorporated a mechanistic model of the visit appropriate only to certain specialties, defined as 'simple' or 'algorithmic' by practitioners. In fact the following comments, by a specialty Chief, suggest that templates were not used *at all* by most clinicians:

Very few people were really using templates. GYN were using them because it's a highly specialised group. It's great for the exam, the history, when you're documenting things like last menstrual period; how frequent are your periods, do you have bleeding in between: really discrete data. As opposed to, 'Doc, I'm tired, I don't feel well today.' Or 'I got a little bit of chest pain. I get a little short of breath.' Very subjective concepts: as opposed to, 'Gimme the date; gimme the number of days.'

A similar view was expressed by a paediatrician:

I'm a paediatrician, so most of my things are single acute problems, although I do have multiple chronic patients; and we don't use templates. I don't think anybody in this clinic uses templates except for well-child visits. They're useless and they're a waste of time and it takes too much time. So what most of us do for the chronic problems – and [another] Clinic taught us this – is that you just list all of your problems and then you just cut and paste from the previous visit and then just change it and save it.

And I think that was really disappointing. We thought 'Wow, this is gonna be great!' And the way they were set up, you couldn't just click on something; if you wanted to free-text you had to click six different buttons, and there were a lot of keystrokes that made it harder. And they didn't help us; they didn't help me make any decisions – there wasn't any decision support.

Care process innovation

Having seen some of the problems, did CIS lead to or support any care process innovation or redesign in Hawaii? Due to the intensity of their workload, and how some defined quality of care, clinics using CIS were severely challenged by the implementation. Yet, paradoxically, some respondents reported that CIS was a spur to innovation. Apparently, this was necessity being the mother of invention, especially in response to the extra time burden imposed on clinicians. Such innovations tended to take the form of experiments in redesigning the visit, or 'workarounds' to circumvent inconvenient features of the software. All but one respondent reported that CIS significantly slowed down the work of physicians, who had compensated by working through lunchtime, leaving work later, ceasing to see 'overloads' (patients without appointments), and reducing social contact with colleagues.

Within customary practice styles, there appears to have been little slack to absorb the additional time burden of working with CIS. Consequently, users, and the region generally, had been forced to recognise a need to redesign how they delivered care to members. Their need to question the sacred cow of the personal visit reverberated with published Institute of Medicine and Institute of Health Improvement reports which questioned the assumed requirement for face-to-face visits in all cases ('The visit is not the visit'). As a result, a growing number of experiments were underway in Hawaii Kaiser Permanente to resolve the contradiction between longer appointments and maintaining and improving access. These included MD telephone triage, group consultations and improvements in chronic disease management. The broad aim was to offer alternative methods of providing care, so that all of those patients who really wanted and needed a clinic visit got one, whilst others could avail themselves of more convenient, timely, and no less effective modes of care for their situation.

E-conversion

Exposure to CIS had helped to convert a significant mass of Hawaii Kaiser Permanente practitioners to the principle of e-health. (The Hope at the bottom of Pandora's Box?) A gradient of belief in the possibilities that e-health would offer was found, but several respondents in positions of influence had, in the words of one member of one implementation team, simply, 'Got it':

To me, probably the most exciting thing that happened in CIS is that there are pockets of people who have got it: who've said, 'This is not just a way to document my chart: it's a totally new way of taking care of patients.' That's catching and the tele-health thing with the doctor on the phone is now in three or four sites.

In terms of specific functions provided by CIS, all the physicians interviewed were convinced of the advantages of an electronic system, even if their CIS experience had been frustrating in many ways. As one Chief explained, the online patient record in particular removed a considerable burden of uncertainty and guesswork from the physician concerning a member's previous care, and its value was noticed keenly whenever the system went down:

Productivity, managing our workflow, our caseload is still a problem. It's much slower for us than paper. It isn't just the notes: it's just using the whole system. But we don't regret being among the first to implement. When it goes down we are all unhappy, all of us: staff, nurses, doctors. It's so much better than paper.

It used to be so frustrating that somebody got seen first at an outlying clinic, and now they're seeing you for follow-up, or they are not better and you have no idea what they did. And you'd have to try and piece together from lab and X-ray and medication, and this and that: 'OK, well, he must have done so-and-so' – you're just guessing. Now, all you have to do is pull up the note: you can know what your RN did, or talked about the day before, or a week before, whatever the case may be. You can read what your colleague did last month. All the information is at your fingertips and everything is documented now.

MD telephone triage

As one Chief reported, relative to MD telephone triage, CIS's online patient record made alternative appointments viable:

We were able to start to do the MD triage, where, since the charts are available, the patient can call in the morning and, instead of having to be seen, maybe we can take care of it over the phone. It's helped open up appointments, and the patients like it because they don't have to come in.

Even the negative pressures could be positively interpreted when they revealed weaknesses and absurdities enshrined in custom and practice, as another speciality Chief related:

To my mind some things are the fault of the IBM system, but in many ways it's kind of a mixed blessing because it really showed a fault in our system, in which our automatic response was: patient has a problem? The doctor has to see you. If someone called in, the Medical Assistant would tell them – I could overhear her say, 'Oh no, the doctor will have to see you. I know you've had this sinusitis every year, but the doctor will still have to see you.' You know, we all said, 'Do we have to do this? I mean I know the guy, he knows sinusitis. I mean it's like a lady with UTI [urinary tract infection], once you've had one it's not too tricky to figure out it's come back!'

The same Chief explained how MD telephone triage actually works:

Basically, there's a group of us that will pitch in and we will talk to patients on the phone. And we have a protocol for which patients would be appropriate to send to us. We have some age limits; we have some illness type markers – if they're having cold-type symptoms to pass it our way and such. And the receptionists do our screening. So the receptionist will get the call, they'll offer, 'Would you like to talk to a doctor on the phone, who'll talk to you within an hour and possibly could help you out without you having to come in?' And the majority of patients are thrilled with it. So because they've spoken to a doctor the scope of practice issue is addressed as well; because the doctor could make a diagnosis over the phone, which the nurse wouldn't be allowed to do. And it's timely. They are not going to send us patients having fevers of 105, and crushing chest pain, [but] by saving inappropriate appointments, it then allows us, with our more limited appointment schedule, to get the people [in] who we need to get in to be seen.

Automation, integration or transformation?

Respondents were asked if they thought CIS implementation had merely automated care processes or transformed them more radically. Opinions were mixed: some felt that automation had been the norm and that the true potential to revolutionise healthcare had been grasped only lightly, as this clinic manager observed:

With CIS the tendency has been to automate rather than redesign care processes. So it's standardised a lot of stuff and improved our efficiency with forms and so on. It's automated what we were doing, but we still need to take a look at access and how we deliver care, because it hasn't cut the time of the visit.

But now we are asking if we need to look at the visit itself differently. And so the healthcare teams are listening to the IOM report and Don Berwick's issue that the visit is not the visit. We are here for the healing relationship. And that can occur not just with the visit, but with a phone call, with email.

Another clinic manager observed a tendency for users to become fixated on CIS functions, instead of viewing them as tools to support practice innovation:

CIS is not the important thing, it's what you do with it, how you use it as a tool to support your practice. In some areas it was like an add-on thing. We were trying to integrate it into our daily work as just one more tool.

Other respondents thought that assimilation of CIS into practice styles remained a major challenge, as one clinic manager related:

What I hear from some providers is: 'I need help in integrating this tool into my practice: I need a coach. Because I was successful, I had my routine, I knew how the visit was going to go. And now this alters the dynamic, the time, whatever. And so I need to go through the visit differently maybe.'

Several respondents envisaged a very different kind of e-health delivery system. One Chief felt that Kaiser Permanente's criteria for excellence were too modest, even complacent, in the context of Hawaii's highly competitive market:

Hawaii is the best region as regards chronic care management: but my feeling is that these comparisons are too internal, and you are only comparing yourself to Kaiser in Georgia or Kaiser in Colorado. Maybe you should be comparing yourself to Queen's Hospital down the street, or Mililani. Or maybe you shouldn't even look at your competitors. Maybe you should look at, 'Well, how good can you really be?'

And my personal bias is that [...] I think there's more that we could do for our patients; I think there are better ways that we could take care of our patients. I don't think that the current way that we take care of patients with care based on visits, and visits documented on a paper record, I think we pretty much have reached the limits of how good that can get you and I don't think that's good enough. I think the electronic medical record is a useful thing that could possibly allow you to break through those limits.

I personally felt that my goal was not to give as good care as I gave before. My goal was to give great care. Why is it defined that good care is seeing 25 patients in a day? That's not good care. Maybe good care is seeing 12 patients in a day but you're serving more people in different ways because you have the information, or you're emailing them or talking to them, or you know what's going on with their life, or we as a team with all of our eyes are able to look at what's happening with that patient. Much more reliable than just requiring docs to remember everything and do everything. And so you need a different tool to do that.

A senior administrator was more sanguine about one large clinic's experience of CIS:

Internal medicine physicians found that they could not get back to seeing their 25 patients a day, because internal medicine involves multiple organs/illnesses and they have to write a lot. So they started at first to blame it on CIS. They said, 'CIS has made us less efficient.' And then pretty soon they said, 'You know, it's not CIS, it's really our care delivery system and the way that we provide care for the patients. There are better ways to do this than a face-to-face visit. We don't really need to do that. We could talk to them on the phone, we could do email. There are ways of relating to the patient other than by seeing them.'

First, because the relationship is important, you have to establish that relationship. But once established they already have trust and confidence in you. That is what relationships provide: trust and confidence. Once you have that there are so many alternative ways to provide for the patient's need, instead of telling them, 'Come in for a 15 minute appointment.' We set it up that way; we set up the whole system to do that.

Because doctors are not paid by the visit, because we are prepaid, we don't have to think about that. And if it is more efficient it's better, so we have a very great incentive to look at this in a very different way. So if nothing else, through all this pain that we went through with CIS, the physicians came to that conclusion, which is dynamite, this is gold to me. And now the physician leadership is really looking at that and we are going to make those radical changes within the delivery system.

At the same time, an Institute of Medicine Report came out and said, 'We all need to change the way that we provide care to patients.' So we looked at that and said, 'God, that's what they've been saying!' We just didn't realise it from our end, I mean not to the extent that we realise it now, because CIS forced us to do that. So in some ways it happened at the right time for us, even though we went through the pain of all of that stuff.

Unless the physicians take ownership of the care delivery system and take a leadership role, it ain't gonna work. Because if I went and said that we have to redesign the care delivery system – and I'm not a physician – people wouldn't listen. Only when the physicians feel that they need to make the change is the change going to happen. And so now we have this great potential to change the delivery system with Epic, which provides all the tools.

So on one side you have the tools, and on the other side you got the people who are ready to do that. So it's sort of like: forget about CIS – but CIS really did us a favour in getting us to this point. It's kind of like we are going to revolutionise the healthcare system. Epic's vision with an integrated product, and we an integrated healthcare system: the marriage is just perfect. Because nobody else can do this except us as an integrated system.

CIS in context: one among many tools

Previous extracts confirm that CIS was not implemented in a national policy vacuum. Calls to redesign the visit in the US (the *appointment* in the UK) in reports by the Institutes of Medicine and Health Improvement had been disseminated widely in Kaiser Permanente. As Sidney Garfield had told the Monterey Conference in 1960, IT innovation is but one important factor in the larger context of ideas and proposals concerning quality improvement in healthcare; a context in which different factors might have cumulative effects on attitudes and opinions, as well as, or instead of, actions.[72] One Chief remarked:

If you look at the Institute of Medicine's report, all that CIS did was to uncover the fact that our system was not able to function and we weren't able to fix it by working harder – because we certainly tried that. [...] We tried to say, 'OK, we're gonna just come in earlier, we're gonna go home later' and we still couldn't fix it. In retrospect, what we needed to do is rethink how we practise medicine.

Another Chief referred to the previous innovation of medical assistants (MAs), which he considered had contributed to the standardisation of care processes. The MA works between exam rooms and therefore to some extent standardises different clinicians' idiosyncratic practices. This mediating role (by the most junior upon the most senior members of the clinical staff) also paved the way to standardise other practices in preparation for CIS:

Suddenly we have three people [MAs] who are significant to the functioning of the department, who cross all boundaries. They see all of the surgeons' patients in different exam rooms and so they've started to standardise the processes, just because they're there. And if you want them to be there, then the MA has to do certain things: rooms have to be set up in a standard way; and the discharge has to be standardised. CIS didn't really do much.

Thus, innovation in the organisation and delivery of care was not wholly dependent on IT, which should be seen as a contributory factor to a more general trend towards improvement and innovation. This was also shown by the introduction of team-based care in some clinics, as part of a policy introduced prior to CIS:

Our focus for this coming year is going to be on access to primary care. What can we do to improve access? One way is to have group clinics. Instead of making one appointment and then another appointment where you say the same thing, you try to get all the team members in one appointment. So you have the dietician, the nutritionist, clinical diabetes educator, clinical pharmacist, physician, nurse, nurse practitioner, so they're all there with the members.

Thus e-healthcare was not seen as an end in itself. The key question seeming to exercise most respondents was how an EMR could be used as one among many tools to improve services to Kaiser Permanente members – preferably without killing Kaiser Permanente employees in the process.

But if Hawaii Kaiser Permanente practitioners felt under greater time pressure due to CIS, longer visits were seen by one Chief as potentially beneficial:

Maybe CIS takes longer because we take better care of the patient and we're doing more for the patient. So maybe it should take longer. At least if we take better care of the patients we'll feel better about what we do. So as long as the electronic patient record is a good system and doesn't have a lot of inbuilt frustration, maybe that slowing down process is a good thing for the patient and for the provider.

We actually had that discussion. That, OK, maybe we don't want to go back to what we were doing before, the number of patients that we were seeing before, because it was not good care. We were just running 'em through, putting band-aids on them and not really taking care of them. And so by it time-limiting us, so that we can't put all these extra patients on our schedule, it's kind of better actually. Although it's not better for the 20 patients who are calling that can't get an appointment. So our day isn't so bad anymore, but front desk is having a really hard time.

Was CIS a spur to innovation? Although there is no simple answer to that question, it did appear that, within an already dynamic context, CIS had a significant positive influence on Kaiser Permanente's aspirations in some important respects, as one Chief remarked:

What we're talking about – the bigger picture – is not about using CIS, that's not our goal. Our goal is to move to an electronic medical record. There are different ways of thinking and interacting.

Other benefits of CIS implementation

The electronic medical record

The ability to refer to an up-to-date electronic medical record convinced many respondents of the actual and potential advantages of 'going electronic'. This assessment appeared to outweigh negative factors which might have discouraged users from computerised systems, as even CIS with all its shortcomings was preferred to paper. One Chief noted:

I don't think any of us want to go back to a paper chart. The advantages of having

> *a computerised record that's easily accessible are profound. We get a lot of phone calls; we do a lot of cross-coverage [now] we have the data at our fingertips.*

Another Chief referred to the cumulative nature of these benefits:

> *One of the true benefits of an electronic medical record isn't from what you're putting in at the time; it's down the road, the investment that you're making. And the longer a clinic is on CIS, the greater the benefit. So I get a phone call, I pull up the chart, I see the previous notes; I see all the things that you imagine are the advantages of an electronic medical record.*
>
> *Putting information in is not particularly easy with CIS; and getting the lab results and dealing with that is not particularly easy with CIS. But having access to the information; being able to take care of the patient with the information there, rather than being frustrated because the chart is at a clinic or en route.*

One Chief enumerated the potential benefits of CIS in terms of legibility, codification and outcome evaluation. It appeared that only legibility had been realised. Codification remained problematic. And using CIS to evaluate health outcomes and contribute to the evidence database had not been achieved at all:

> *Number one is legibility. I think there is a tremendous problem in trying to read anybody's note. Numbers two and three are codification, and the establishment of a research database.*
>
> *When you are moving quickly and when your charges are not created by the amount you document, you write less and less. And you get two or three line notes that don't say very much to anybody else. They may say a lot to you, but an internist cannot look at that note and have any clue about what's going on. Being able to go back and utilise that data and say: 'Can we improve healthcare? Can we actually take what we've done and tell if we've made any difference?'*
>
> *If you took X million members and decided: OK we're going to look at prostate cancer and we are going to look at 100 variables, that you collect anyway – the patient's age, do they have diabetes, heart disease, what medications are they on; how big is their prostate, how many units of blood do they get transfused during surgery, how many biopsies did they do? If we can go back and eliminate enough of the confounding variables, we may actually come up with an answer, even though it's a retrospective study, that says: 'This treatment is better than this because we have a cohort of 400 000,' instead of, 'I did 32 patients with me and my partner over the last 12 years and here's what we did.' I think with Kaiser Permanente's size you have enough patients to do that with virtually any disease process. From what I heard when I first came here, this was the whole reason for the project. We were going to get all this data that we could make healthcare decisions on.*

Accountability

CIS was perceived to have made clinicians more accountable, in several ways. As preparation for CIS they had had to account for their practice procedures to their peers and teams, and perhaps even to themselves. CIS required physicians to record and sign-off on all decisions and actions on a time and date stamped record accessible to other users. Responses to these demands varied. In addition to general improvements in the openness and reliability of care, CIS was perceived by one member of the implementation team to have helped clarify and rationalise roles and responsibilities at the affected sites:

> I think it forces you to be very explicit about how you do things. I think we've seen more sharing of responsibility: for having nurses do follow-up phone calls, and follow-up on certain types of results; and understanding what an MA specifically can do for you and can't do for you; and shifting some work off the physician to the others. And improving the coverage system when people were away: how do you handle results? That used to be informal: somebody would just throw it on a desk. Now you have to be very explicit – if Joe is away, who's going look at his results? The computer's got to know who to send it to.

Another effect was to turn physicians into more conscientious *authors*. Previously, notes had been written mainly for their own guidance; now they were aware of a large potential audience. One informant said that CIS had forced him to record his actions better. He knew that he should have set a higher standard for himself before, but had not been under any external pressure to do so:

> No question in my mind, it's forced me to be more organised, more accountable – and that's the hard part, it's the accountability part, where we see a lab and we sign off on it. Everyone knows when you looked at it; when you signed off for it, what your plans are. Previously it was easy to look at a sheet of paper with the lab report and decide what you're going to do, and it [was] a little bit nebulous. But now the accountability is there for everybody to see. I'm using it in the terms of a good way, as something good. It's forced me to do what I should have been doing all along, but which I haven't been.

This view was supported by members of the implementation team, who attributed improvements in clinician accountability not only to the bureaucratic demands of the software but to a change in the mindset of users, who were more engaged with the wider professional network that CIS opened to them:

> Somehow it has changed the psyche of people documenting, and they are very much more aware of what they are putting in the chart, something we never really quite anticipated. When you see the electronic signatures on the charts, people sit up. It's almost like they didn't really care about what they wrote on paper, but now that it's electronic and people can read everything, you can't hide behind, 'Well that scribble says this'. It has really opened people's eyes and made them more careful. It's legible, attributable, accountable.

One implementation team member noted that CIS had improved the accountability of medical practitioners in the sense of submitting the hitherto private space of the exam room to a new visibility:

> It has sort of opened up the doors to the exam room. I don't think there was that openness before CIS. I think one of the things that putting in the computer allowed us to do, is to talk more about what the workflow looks like. Before, the physicians wholly defined the workflow.
>
> As there are limitations to every tool, in some ways the application [CIS] defined the workflow, and then all the other players got to say: 'Well it would work better for me if we did it this way.' So it allowed us to have some discussion about things that we really didn't discuss before.

This new visibility finally pushes physicians to the periphery of Bentham's Panopticon,[22] a place previously occupied only by the patients and medical menials.* Who then is the unseen observer occupying the central tower of Bentham's model? That role has been generalised – and further virtualised – into anyone who can log on to the CIS system to call up its records. Note that, in close accord with the panoptic model, it is the observer's virtual, unseen and unconfirmed presence – not that of an actual visible observer, 'who' commands the compliance of physicians to a higher standard of record keeping. Hence we can also see that the social impact of CIS, and of new IT in healthcare more widely, is partly a politico-administrative apparatus designed to make professionals more visible and accountable to the corporation and, perhaps, to society.

It is indeed remarkable that physicians have evaded an institutional principle that much of the rest of society has obeyed for so long, and how successful their rearguard actions have been and continue to be. In a sense, Paul Starr's acclaimed history of American medicine is an account of its struggle to retain its craft status against the forces of modernisation.[76] It is a reasonable hypothesis, moreover, that conservative physicians' implicit understanding of this very implication of new IT in healthcare – the new light it shines into their private offices and arcane practices – would inform their resistance to its adoption and implementation, in Hawaii Kaiser Permanente as elsewhere.

Decision making

Implementation team members reported that the complex and ambiguous experience of CIS implementation had yielded transferable skills, which might be overlooked by a simplistic assessment of CIS as a failed project. For example, one significant outcome of implementation had been the creation of an infrastructure for leadership and communication. This had improved decision-making capability across clinics and specialties:

> *The Chiefs have not been organised around a project like this before. There are a lot of projects always happening but usually it's kind of like, 'How's this going*

---

*English social philosopher Jeremy Bentham proposed a technically efficient design for prisons consisting of a circular arrangement of cells surrounding a high tower. The structure allowed every inmate to be observed by a single person in the tower, who remained invisible to them. Nor could inmates see one another. Being uncertain as to whether they were being observed, inmates would have to assume constant surveillance. Bentham named this design the Panopticon. Michel Foucault proposes the Panopticon as a model of the disciplinary technologies based on mass-surveillance that grew to dominate Western society from the late eighteenth century. The penitentiary at Stateville, Illinois, for instance, was built on the panoptic model. The Panopticon is really a refinement of earlier systems of visibility, such as simple segregation between sick and healthy in times of plagues, and the rectilinear arrangement of schools, barracks and hospital wards. Computer networks operate in a similar way to the Panopticon by allowing the decisions of dispersed operators to be monitored centrally and remotely. Foucault identified in panopticism a psycho-social principle: one internalises the rule of surveillance to become one's own supervisor or warder – the soul, as Foucault puts it, which is the pilot of the body. In the present context an EMR permits the remote assessment of inputs by identified operators, who can never be certain whether they are being watched. When Hawaii Kaiser Permanente physicians adapted their note making to CIS, they began to behave like the inmates of a Panopticon. The fact that some agreed with this increased accountability confirms that their warder-consciences were already aware of their lack of rigour. They were even glad to be coerced in exchange for an easier conscience.

to affect my department?' This project made them come together and say, 'OK, we have to make some big decisions, we have to make policy decisions. Who's going to dictate, who's going to not dictate: we have a chance to change that policy. And we can't make it different for ortho and medicine and paeds, it all has to be the same.' So we put a structure together where we met with them around policy decisions, project-wide for the whole region, and that was something new. For instance we have the Chiefs now to problem solve. Getting them together in the beginning was challenging but now they have regular meetings and they know the kinds of decisions to be made. The right decisions are going to the right groups. There is an organisation of managers, an organisation of supervisors, so that's the kind of infrastructure that is a lot more organised than we were at the beginning.

One Chief agreed that the CIS implementation process had yielded generic benefits transcending the specific application:

The system was too rigid and clunky. But we do have the infrastructure set up for it – so that's nice: and now if we can overlay a better system on top of it then it might work well.

And a member of the implementation team thought that the implementation process marked a qualitative advance in computer literacy:

There tends to be a lack of trust in the challenging group, so that after an unsuccessful implementation…and some people would tell you that we've had several unsuccessful implementations. I, on the other hand, would put a spin on it and say that where we've gone from very limited computer literacy, as an organisation, to one that expects to be able to walk around and use any one of these tools, has been a huge and positive journey.

Interagency communication

One Chief noted that CIS had supported better communication between Hawaii Kaiser Permanente and other health and social care organisations:

I think there's better transparency, which is good. I would never really have thought about giving a copy of my note to care homes. I do that routinely now. In the past I would write my own note in the chart and then I would write a very abbreviated note in the care home chart, that they needed to maintain their accreditation. But now I actually just give them the entire note. I print out a copy of my note.

We do the same thing when we use consultants outside Kaiser. It's a lot easier to give them the documentation, because they don't have to worry about not being able to read it. There aren't pieces attached that, when you Xerox it, may not be appropriate. I actually let the patient carry it with them to see their consultant. All of these things I don't think we would have done earlier. It never dawned on me to do it.

An implementation team member reflected on the wider implications of changes wrought by CIS. One issue related to the viability of Kaiser Permanente as an organisation that had always swum against the current of fee-for-service healthcare in the US, and raised the (mainly Republican) taboo of 'socialised medicine':

Even within Kaiser as an organisation, I think there are still areas that you could probably describe as a collection of private practices. And the implementation in Colorado greyed those lines and made it more homogenous. And then as they tried to implement CIS across the regions, that greyed the lines even further and made it even more homogenous.

We used to talk about how this was going to change Kaiser as an organisation in ways that nobody understands yet. In some cases it's taken nearly 10 years, but I think we are starting to see it now in that the organisation is actually welcoming conversations about, 'Let's standardise our intake process; let's standardise other processes and procedures.' Because they recognise that it's to our members' benefit not to see large variations in healthcare services, and the way healthcare is administered. And it's advantageous to us as an organisation, because now we can predict and control costs much better if we know how everybody is doing it across the board.

But maybe it's just setting a baseline, which should have been there for a long time anyway. You could probably take it to the far extreme and say that it's approaching socialised medicine. I don't think so, but I've heard those comments before in some of the hallway conversations that we've had: that this was moving us further and faster down the road towards the concept of socialised medicine, where everybody is doing exactly the same thing.*

I don't sign on to that philosophy. But it's easy to see how someone could think that you could walk into any Kaiser facility and any exam room and, if you didn't look at the weather outside, you might not even know what city you were in, because the services are the same, the buildings are the same. It takes corporate medicine to a whole new level that nobody had contemplated before. Is that a bad thing? I don't know. Is it something that's going to allow Kaiser as an organisation to be more responsive to the needs of our community, the needs of our members, the needs of the industry? Maybe: and maybe our death knell too. I don't know. I don't know where it's going to go yet.

Quality

One implementation team member was adamant that some of the changes brought about by the implementation of CIS were both beneficial and necessary in view of tighter constraints imposed on healthcare organisations by Federal government:

I would venture that much of what was previously done was not acceptable. But we got away with it. I don't mean that people were deliberately trying to do things, but that this was how they coped with, you know, 'My panel of patients is getting bigger: I need more time. So if I'm seeing somebody I'll do that three line summary.' But it may not pass muster when it comes to what the Federal government is going to require from us.

---

*Socialised medicine in this context appears to be defined as the enemy of consumer sovereignty, choice supposedly exercised through the market system; component myths of the American dream, enshrined in public opinion and antitrust law. And yet, beneath the consumerist ideology there is a very real suspicion of monopolistic control in the USA.

So I tend to see it in a different perspective in that CIS requires it, but it's always been required. We got sloppy. I hesitate even to say that word about these hard-working people that have all this heart for their members, but we just didn't do the work we needed to do. Chart audits were potentially very poor.

One Chief agreed with this assessment:

It really identified areas where we had been lax, to my mind, or areas where we hadn't really thought it through. In that sense I think we do a much better job.

The visit is not the visit

As well as face-to-face, doctor–patient interaction, CIS was designed to affect many care-related processes including coding, billing, ordering, results, etc. In fact, relatively little attention was reportedly given to the implications of CIS for the visit itself. How would physicians cope with serving system and member together? How would they divide their time between the two? Which CIS tasks could be performed before, during or after the visit? How would CIS affect the socio-clinical dynamic of the visit? How would patients interpret this novel situation? The absence of specific attention to these effects suggests a general assumption that CIS would be assimilated into practices without disrupting established styles and rhythms. This is not to say that these issues were not addressed, at least at some implementation sites, but that they were not expected to be especially problematical. Actually, they were.

Indeed, the implementation team noted a wide variation in responses to the arrival of the 'Cisco Kid'* in the consulting room:

It varies depending on the person. There are people who do a lot more shared decision making and sharing of information because the computer is in there. Somehow it's just easier to show people a screen than a paper chart.

Then there are people who are struggling so hard to get everything in the computer that their members are telling us: 'They talk to the computer; they don't talk to me anymore.' And that's in spite of trying to introduce the concept of communicating with the computer [as a tool for patient–provider communication].

There are some people who are intuitive communicators and they love having the computer in there and they thrive on it; and there's other people that they are just going: [mimics stiff posture] and their hands are tense and they are typing and they are staring right at the screen.

---

*CIS was referred to as 'the Cisco Kid' by two pairs of respondents. We deduced that the nickname conveyed an interesting nest of meanings. The prefix 'Cis-' conceives CIS as a third party in the visit; while the suffix '-co' denotes a *corporate* presence; and a reference to the San Francisco Bay Area, where Kaiser Permanente HQ is located. The implications include that CIS was viewed somewhat ironically as (1) a benevolent digital stranger sent to deliver them from an analogical dark age, and (2) an intrusion by the corporate world (of IBM and possibly northern California region). It is unlikely that any of those propositions were true or false *per se*. The Cisco Kid label had both mythic and derisory functions: to render the complexity and contingency of decision processes higher up the organisation comprehensible; to satirise those responsible; and to personify what would otherwise remain a diffuse and hard to apprehend technology. This process can be summarised as *anthropocentric*: in this instance the complex, lofty and remote rendered human and fallible

Unsurprisingly, doctors familiar with home PCs tended to have less difficulty integrating CIS into their practices. For some others it seemed to pose a challenge to their professional pride and identity, as another CIS team member commented:

> *A lot of the younger docs, who are used to talking to their kids and being on the Internet at the same time, are cool with it, they have a natural ability. Some of the guys who are my age or older took pride in the fact they don't type.*
>
> *So does it come between us, as we have this sometimes very intimate conversation about what your concerns are? Or is it a tool that gives you more confidence in my ability?*

The same informant thought the e-literate group a majority and some had found that using CIS as a visual aid in the visit had enhanced their relationships with members:

> *Some people have actually found that it's been a real tool to improve their relationships with their patients. I think the majority of the doctors do show their patients what's on the screen. It's sharing. You know, people experience and learn in different ways. So to actually see it on the screen, to see your lab results: you [the patient] may be a more visual person, so it may stick with you more to see that, or to see trends.*

Although no Kaiser Permanente members (subscribers or patients) were interviewed in this study, a few respondents reported positive feedback on CIS by patients, as a senior administrator noted:

> *Exit interviews tell us that our members like this. They think that we're smarter doctors, they think that we care more about them when we can show them these things on a screen that reflect customised care for them.*

A paediatrician reported that child patients were impressed by doctors' use of CIS in their visits:

> *Some of them like it; a lot of them think it's kinda neat. For the kids I can pull up the growth chart and I can show it to them, and they think that's kinda cool. The fact they can go to another clinic and their chart will be there in the ER, that's a plus for them. I haven't had any patient not like it.*

However, one CIS team member was more sceptical, interpreting patients' responses to CIS as relatively uninformed and therefore of limited significance. The more e-literate members tended to view CIS as a generic sign of progress:

> *I think almost every provider experienced in some way the potential of what it could eventually be, in terms of a visit where I can go in and show you your labs, and it's telling me we need to look at your [...] And I think patients as a whole were very excited by it, because they felt from experience, 'you'll know me', and the potential for them, 'Maybe I can email you; or maybe I can get some of my answers by not coming in.' I think the Internet-savvy patients were excited by the image of progress; of the flat screens in the exam room; of bringing healthcare into the twenty-first century. So I think everybody was excited about the potential.*

Chronic disease management

All respondents were asked if CIS had impacted on chronic disease management. Most referred to the Population Care Registry (PCR), an existing electronic application, which provided a limited population focus. One clinic had begun to use PCR and CIS together to try to improve the management of members with chronic conditions, as a clinician explained:

> We are starting to do a little bit more patient care management, and I don't think we could have done it with paper charts because we would have had to pull maybe 40, 50 charts.
>
> But we meet in this room; we've got two computers going: somebody's laptop is in with PCR running, and then we've got CIS – so if there's a question we can just pull it up. And we've got our list of CHF [congestive heart failure] patients, or diabetes patients and we just go through them and see what medications they're on and everything like that. We can take care of a lot of patients in a short period of time. So it's kind of a project that started this year and I don't think we could have done it without an electronic medical record.

A CIS team member wrote to describe how that clinic's innovation in chronic disease management worked in more detail:

> I think it's really exciting: because now, for instance, one of our clinics, that we just deployed late last year, they are using it as a tool to manage their diabetics and their heart failure patients; and it's not 'CIS', it's a tool for their population management. The clinic has organised provider 'teams' to manage a panel of chronic patients, and utilises the electronic record as a reference tool in their process. The team is made up of an MD, NP [nurse practitioner], RN, MA, CDE [certified diabetic educator] and receptionist. They meet once a week for approximately two hours. During this time, they complete a 'case review' of approximately 40 patients identified by PCR. In the conference room where they meet, they access PCR, CIS and Kaiser Permanente mainframe systems to reference information when making clinical decisions.
>
> They are finding that CIS has allowed them to be more efficient in this case review process, in that they are not dependent on 'flipping' through pages of a paper chart to search for the latest information. Also, documentation can occur immediately. They have started this process with CHF patients and will soon begin to include a review of their diabetic patients. We are assisting the clinic with the documentation of this case review process, [and] to address requests for start up information from other Healthcare Teams who are on CIS.

But other informants thought that, far from improving it, CIS had diverted their attention from chronic disease management. This was particularly the case for hard-pressed internists (who have most interest in chronic disease), as one Chief had found relative to the controversial templates:

> I'm sure that dermatology or ophthalmology or even ortho would fly with it. But internal medicine, where you're dealing with three or four chronic diseases atop an acute problem: it became burdensome. And as we made suggestions to improve things they were just ignored and their time schedule went on its merry way.

Another internist found that CIS reduced the time available for chronic disease management via the PCR:

> *In the one year that we've used CIS, I'd say that it's had a negative impact. Because it diverted so much of my mental capacity towards, 'Get the note done, get the note done. Not enough time, hurry up: get the note done!' that I didn't have time to stop and ponder, 'What else needs to be done?' And CIS wasn't advanced enough to provide us with those reminders or those flow charts that would facilitate care.*
>
> *The PCR had chronic disease reminders on it. When CIS came I had my nurse stop printing out the PCR because I would never look at it anyway. I was too busy flipping between screens just trying to make it through the clinic visit. So I think there has been a negative impact. But I understand there would have been a positive impact if we had stuck it out long enough. But how long is long enough? In this day and age, they are telling us two or three years: that's unacceptable, that's way too long.*

Other lessons learned from implementing CIS

Several informants reflected on what Kaiser Permanente had learned from the global experience of trying to implement CIS. Members of the implementation team reported most of the lessons, though one spoke for physicians:

> *Looking after the best interests of the organisation means looking after the best interests of the physicians. They would say, 'In order for CIS to work well, I have to work well' – 'I' being a physician. That's a hard thing for us to say because nobody wants to benefit personally: it's always the higher organisational team goal that's important. We've all been trained, we've all been indoctrinated that way and we all follow that very well.*

This suggests that user-friendliness to physicians is a *sine qua non* of success with any EMR, and that self-interest is contrary to the norms of Hawaii Kaiser Permanente culture. This is a double bind: if the system does not work for physicians it does not work for the organisation. But physicians are reluctant to report that deficiency for fear of seeming self-centred, so the organisation does not find out about it. One lesson from this could be that Hawaii Kaiser Permanente was not the best place to test a beta version. Some among the Hawaii staff were too polite to pick fault, preferring to be agreeable, and either struggle quietly on with CIS, or just not use it. We revisit this issue in more detail under 'Organisational culture' below.

Another lesson concerned the amount of preparation needed prior to actual implementation:

> *I think the biggest lesson I've learned across these various project teams and deployments is not to underestimate the pre-work that needs to be done.*

And there were more general acknowledgements that the CIS project had been a profitable educational experience:

> *People seem to have learned a lot. Clinicians seem to have learned a lot about what they were doing before, through analysing their processes of care as a preparation for being trained on CIS. All your workflows are affected by converting to an electronic system, so understanding actually what you're doing and making some*

changes to adapt to the new system, it's a very educational process, a team building process.

Finally, one member of the CIS team noted that its implementation had provided opportunities to learn about and improve interregional relations within Kaiser Permanente:

> *I think it became apparent how difficult that [relationship] was, and how many different attitudes in the organisation had to change. I think we learned a lot organisationally. We learned a lot about what our limitations are; what we do well and what we don't do well as an organisation. I think all the regions learned how to work together much better; became less separate little empires and more aware that we needed to act in concert together and not in dissonance. And I think an awful lot of that came about as a function of attempting to install CIS.*

Summary of reported experience of CIS

The overall impression of the data presented in this chapter is somewhat complex and ambiguous. Already we begin to see how inadequate success and failure are as summary judgements on the implementation; how unhelpful it would be to draw premature and inappropriate conclusions in terms of triumph or defeat: not only across the region, but also for specific sites and individuals. We began by noting a 14-month delay in software delivery, yet this is hardly surprising. Experience repeatedly demonstrates the challenges faced in delivering innovative projects on time. Perhaps the real failure, if there is one, refers more nearly to an endemic excessive optimism in innovation, a mood that tends to produce unrealistic deadlines, but without which the rate of progress could actually be much slower. People with 'vision', an imprecise but descriptive term, are often different from those with a meticulous mind for planning and logistics. One creates or sees new connections: the other administers their detailed implications. Both are needed, but it is the former type who drives innovation forward by inciting a mood, optimistic and slightly hysterical, within which even the steadiest minds are caught up and persuaded to commit to dates that in more sober moments they know to be unrealistic. If there is a failure here, it is not that driving optimism, but rather a failure to see a repeated pattern of delays to innovations. In this context, one might call for a tempering of optimism, on one hand, and a softening of expectations, on the other. Or we could be shockingly pragmatic and just accept that delays of this sort are likely, if not inevitable.

The product deficiencies reported may have a similar character to delay, insofar as innovation, particularly involving systemic change, inevitably involves trial and error. But the evidence is not so forgiving. To call CIS a turkey is pretty uncompromising. On balance the data suggests that CIS was actually a lousy product. There are two likely causes. Firstly, the architecture of CIS may have been metaphorically designed as a rigid structure of steel and glass, instead of as a flexible 'information superhighway'. Functional inadequacies could be fixed only by making deep structural alterations, whereas a superhighway concept might have produced a system capable of changing flows by switching lanes and signposts. If that explanation fails, as it well might, perhaps the problem lay not so much in the conception of the EMR system *per se*, as in its joint design and construction between Kaiser Permanente and IBM. After all, if neither could understand the other's messages, it isn't hard to see how a monster could have been made between them. Perhaps the key passage here, which we have already seen, is this one:

> *And then there were changes in the product that was delivered that were very unexpected: think 'Non-starts'. It's like: 'You said you were gonna deliver X, you delivered Y, Y can't be worked with. You must go back and redo this to deliver X.'*

The same respondent used the metaphor of Kaiser and IBM *throwing software over a wall to one another*. This image is powerful in suggesting that both entities were trying to describe things to one another that could not be seen or handled in advance of delivery. Supposing product X was interpreted as Y. Clearly the describer of X might not recognise Y when delivered. One can imagine both sides struggling to interpret the messages of the other: physicians describing their clinical needs; IBM staff translating their descriptions into a set of technical functions and a graphical computer interface. If so, it was more than a communication problem: the whole mode of development was misconceived.

The Pandora's Box effect of CIS is one of the most interesting. It suggests that participants were naive about the scale of organisational adjustment that would be required to translate a paper-based healthcare system into computer architecture. As one respondent noted, CIS touched everything. Computerisation is not like doing the same old things but in new offices: everything one does must be analysed and redesigned. This is the difference between mere automation and transformation. Perhaps automation would have worked, but some of the most ardent supporters of 'going electronic' saw it as a means to transforming their healthcare delivery system. Anything less would have been, and was, frustrating. Nowhere is this more apparent than in the perceived loss of flexibility: the need for physicians to enter more data; the loss of verbal orders; the overturning of localised practices of doubtful legitimacy. But as we have also seen, a process of adjustment had been accomplished by many: new protocols; revised roles; the rejection of certain functions (which might well have been returned to and incorporated at a later date). We need to be cautious about all this because our data were collected in a period of transition between CIS and EpicCare. It is ultimately impossible to predict how the implementation of CIS might have rolled out had it been given more time.

Equally interesting and significant is how unexpected innovations occurred in order to cope with intolerable burdens. Whilst we would not prescribe stress and overload as a legitimate managerial tool, there may be lessons to learn here. In extreme situations some people shine. There are probably enough naturally occurring extreme situations in our workaday lives without deliberately adding more. So perhaps the sensible and humane approach would be simulation. What would we do in a hypothetical situation? What would have to be invented?

Finally, we note that, as well as unanticipated innovations, other benefits came from CIS. On the whole, Hawaii Kaiser Permanente saw the future that CIS promised but did not entirely deliver: an up to date health record; more efficient and better exchange of information; improved record keeping and accountability. Paradoxically the failure of CIS to flourish in Hawaii nonetheless yielded some important seeds of success. After the experience, all respondents agreed that they now had a much clearer conception of what a really good EMR would look like.

Chapter 3

Accounting for successes and failures

In Chapter 2 we presented a summary of participants' experiences of CIS in Hawaii Kaiser Permanente. This chapter interprets the interview data from two further perspectives that, whilst superficially different, are actually related in terms of implementation inputs, processes, and outcomes, and which have thus far received little attention in the literature. The first perspective involves a deeper exploration of participants' experiences of CIS implementation in Hawaii Kaiser Permanente. Whilst this qualitative examination should be interesting in itself we have also a more functional aim, which is (secondly) to articulate an immanent critique of the language of 'success and failure' which this nuanced analysis implies. The binary opposition of success and failure is employed routinely in discussing innovations, but, through speaking to participants, we found it to be highly problematic and largely inadequate, except perhaps in the perennially odd and peremptory gloss on organisational life that is executive-speak. Such a simplistic polarisation of complex diachronic phenomena so clearly misses all the nuances, the twists and turns of decision making, as to make sense only as an external administrative judgement of convenience. A good deal of tacit and sometimes open resistance by respondents to categorising their experience of CIS as either success or failure was encountered. This is reasonable as life is hopefully always more complex, interesting and educational than that simple evaluation allows. In this chapter, therefore, we drill down into the data to examine in more detail the decisions made, including the adoption decision, how CIS fared in the Colorado region, and the knotty question of blame. We also consider contextual issues such as organisational culture and leadership in more detail. Then we examine some important aspects of the approach to implementing CIS, including pilot sites, work study, teambuilding, and organisational readiness. Finally in this chapter, we explore in more detail the metaphor of CIS implementation as opening a Pandora's Box of informal organisational and clinical routines; we look at how the implementation team was managed, the time burden imposed on physicians and others, the impact of previous IT innovations, and the phenomena of resistance and conflict, which CIS incited. The overall message in this detailed analysis is that simplistic judgements along the lines of success or failure are actually unhelpful in assessing complex organisational innovation and implementation.

The decision to adopt CIS

The decision to adopt CIS was controversial. Some members of the Hawaii team favoured a different system and had to decide how they should respond if the adoption decision went against them. As one implementation team member observed, it was really a case of Hobson's choice:

> CIS was the third national [IT] project we've implemented. At the time of the selection we had to decide, 'You know it may go against us: what are we gonna do? If they pick the other one [CIS], do we still wanna go first?' And the answer to that was 'Yes', largely based on, I think, everybody felt the need of an electronic medical record. There wasn't any other option. I mean the way our organisation works, 'You either do this, you don't have to do it, but you still pay your share of the cost, whether you do it or not.'

Ironically, as the previous respondent noted, one of the alternative systems considered was ultimately chosen to replace CIS:

> I think they looked at Epic, which was eliminated because it wasn't scalable. And it turns out they are now getting around the scalability issue by multiple instances: a sort of publish and subscribe system for dealing with the different instances. Whether that was technically feasible three, four years ago when the decision was made – I suspect it was. I don't know what happened there, whether they got bad advice. They hired some consultants and that didn't work out very well.

Doubts about the suitability of CIS were confirmed when the software was finally delivered, as one Chief recalled:

> There was a faction of people who felt strongly that CIS was not the best option for us; that it was a mistake to go with CIS. And in retrospect I have to say that they were right. They had looked at other programs; they thought that the functionality of CIS was not state of the art. And so as a clinic Chief I'm heading towards trying to get my staff ready for this and I'm being addressed by people whom I respect, saying, 'This is a mistake: you should do what you need to do to stop this before it goes on.' And I felt very conflicted then.

That feeling of conflict is part of a theme reported more fully later in this chapter.

CIS in Colorado and Hawaii

If Colorado Kaiser Permanente region had been using CIS successfully, why could Hawaii region not do likewise? One reported reason was that Colorado had longer consultation times – a significant difference perceived by Hawaii Kaiser Permanente physicians and systems engineers prior to the adoption decision. One CIS team member recalled:

> See, a number of us went to Colorado, where they had the IBM system [CIS] already in place for a number of years. Some of us came away thinking: 'That's going to be very difficult to implement here.' And so we even went to the extent of having a meeting with the top leaders to voice this opinion. Colorado has 20-minute appointments and we have 15. One of the feelings was that them having 20 minutes gives them the time to do all the necessary documentation, review of labs, and other things associated with the CIS system. Over here, even without CIS, we are already challenged with trying to keep up with the schedule. Physicians

were spending 10 to 11 hours a day even without CIS, so to bring in something else that might lengthen their day even further was very worrisome to them.

The same group saw Epic being used in Northwest region, as one Chief recalled:

We took one trip to Colorado, which had an older version of CIS, and one trip to Northwest, which had Epic – and we really liked this Northwest system, it just looked good. But Colorado had made CIS work and so we were using some of their tools and methods, but some of them wouldn't work in Hawaii. Like, they had a big phone centre, and our philosophy is: no big phone centre. They had physicians who did not have patients: they would be roving physicians on the floor to help support. Whereas we grab our docs and say: 'You will see this patient!' because access is a problem for us.

Hence some respondents had foreseen at least some of the challenges experienced with CIS in Hawaii, as another physician noted:

The real important part is that many of the problems with the IBM-based system could have been foretold. We set up a group called the CIS Workflow Team prior to us even really knowing the system too well, trying to figure out where the problems were going to be and where we'd have to do workarounds, and how we'd have to change our way of thinking and our way of operating. And we pretty much predicted many of the problems that we experienced. Because we're going to document more, there's a price for documentation. The price is you can't see as many patients.

Who was to blame?

Despite their commitment to Kaiser Permanente, most respondents were cautious about blaming IBM (the system vendor) for CIS's failings. One Chief thought the fault lay in the contract between Kaiser Permanente and IBM:

I'm not sure that IBM was really at fault. I think that IBM was just responding to what we were telling them to do. And the advice Kaiser Permanente was giving them was what was handcuffing them. They had no incentive to really reach out and speed things up. As I understand it there was no proprietary contract: it was Kaiser's and Kaiser's only. 'OK, well then we'll just fix what you tell us. Why should we invest a lot of time and energy into making this a world class product if we can't sell it?'

Others echoed the view that the desired changes to CIS were slow and expensive because IBM did not have an interest in marketing the application elsewhere. But other views were expressed on the issue of whether IBM was actually prevented from marketing CIS by the contract. Indeed a mythology had grown up around the contract, in a seeming absence of clear information. Weighing the different views against one another, along with the likely authority of their purveyors, the most plausible account is that Kaiser did *not* prevent IBM from selling CIS on the open market. The problem was that CIS was so specific to Kaiser Permanente that IBM found it to be unmarketable elsewhere. CIS was clearly cumbersome to change even in response to Kaiser Permanente's requirements, let alone those of other potential customers. One implementation team member asserted that, by seeking a bespoke system, Kaiser Permanente had ended up being its own worst customer:

> Because IBM certainly had every intention to market CIS, in fact large efforts were spent to market CIS to other organisations. But the degree of specificity that CIS had to the Kaiser organisation I think made it difficult. It would be such a large price tag to turn around and make CIS what it needed to be for the next organisation, it just wasn't practical. Even though the core components of CIS were well designed, and could be responsive to a business's needs, the GUI [graphical user interface; pronounced 'gooey'] structure and other specifics in the GUI were very specific to Kaiser and how Kaiser does business.

Whatever the relationship between Kaiser Permanente and IBM, the bespoke nature of CIS contributed to its downfall. It was built around a static image of an organisation actually undergoing rapid change. It turned out to be more of a strait-jacket than the lightweight, versatile garment clinicians wanted. As one Chief concluded:

> I think canning CIS was a good thing only because of its inflexibility. I don't know if it was IBM, it might have been our guys. 'Cause a lot of times we blame the outside company when it turns out to be our IT.

According to one implementation team member, the working arrangement between Kaiser Permanente and IBM was ill-conceived:

> I think they really underestimated IBM's ability to handle the technical issues. It was really a problem in system integration, so Kaiser took a lot of the work on itself to put in different components of the system, and we're not a software or systems integration company. I think they underestimated the difficulty in making the transition between OS2 and Windows NT. And I think they didn't understand the difficulty, the cost, the expense of improving the product, and the fact that IBM weren't putting any R&D money into it compared with their competitors.

Noting the flaws in CIS, one Chief speculated that Kaiser Permanente had been blinded by IBM's reputation as a hardware manufacture to its more limited expertise as a software designer:

> I suppose when we think about it, we oughtn't have gone with a company noted for their hardware, to get software from them that was still being made. Because we'd get a version, we'd complain about the version, we'd be told they couldn't fix the version, and that got very frustrating. Then you kept having to learn new versions, so you'd have to unlearn workarounds that you had developed.

As we saw in the previous section, early CIS users in Hawaii found the application slow and inconvenient to use ('clunky'). These flaws were compounded by the high cost of correction. Indeed, the adoption decision was adjudged a bad business decision, as insufficient attention was given to the long-term cost implications for Kaiser Permanente bearing all the development costs of the beta version and all future improvements, as another implementation team member noted:

> Organisationally, we should never have started down this road of trying to build software ourselves. It's extremely expensive – we are the only client funding the entire R&D. It doesn't make any sense. Was anybody thinking a year or two down the road, 'Did we really have the finances to do what we needed to do to make the

trajectory work?' Because if you look at medical software development, there's a trajectory that you have to be on in order to keep up, and we were never funded for that.

Organisational culture

The adoption decision was further complicated by Hawaii Kaiser Permanente's strong aversion to open disagreement and conflict. It was feared that to refuse a request would be interpreted as unfriendly, impolite and confrontational. This cultural norm may not have been fully appreciated by Kaiser Permanente nationally, fostering dysfunctional communication with Hawaii. Whether CIS was technically adequate or inadequate, it functioned poorly in the Hawaiian context, as one member of the CIS team explained:

> *In some ways Hawaii is not a good place to try out a new system because people here will volunteer to be first, but they might not tell you if it wasn't any good. That's why we'll be better off with Epic than with IBM, because with Epic you have got a proven product, whereas with CIS you've got an alpha system. I mean we were making changes at the weekend to implement on Monday. This is not a good place to come out and test new products for development. It's a good place to implement products that are already evolved and known to work well.*

Hawaii Kaiser Permanente culture appeared to be a cultivar of Hawaiian culture. Traditional collective values of friendliness, family and caring for others were consciously promoted, both within the organisation and through the mass media, with the slogan, 'Caring for Hawaii's people like family'. This culture was often contrasted with the US mainland, viewed as impersonal, unfriendly and unconcerned with maintaining supportive relationships.

'Culture,' declared one Chief, 'will eat technology for lunch.' But Kaiser Permanente culture was far from homogeneous: each clinic and specialty had its own locality, linked with different technologies, biological systems, provider personalities, leaders, ethnic mixes, locations, sizes, and numbers of teams. Even so, the importance of defining and adhering to core values to safeguard Kaiser Permanente culture was constantly emphasised.

Kaiser Permanente culture hinges on a concept of the family. Hawaiian culture enshrines certain values, notably – and these may be regarded as their 'holy trinity' – *aloha*, connoting love, warmth, social inclusion, extending oneself to others; *ohana*, denoting strong family ties; and *hanai*, which refers to extending family boundaries beyond kinship. This trinity supports a Hawaiian tendency to adopt biologically unrelated individuals or groups into their families. The beliefs that everyone should be loved and needs a family lead logically to adoption when the perceived need arises. This ethos was often explicitly and proudly invoked by respondents to account for a wide range of behaviour. One regional policy maker described Kaiser Permanente as a huge extended family, including both employees and members:

> *We in Hawaii are kind of the Aloha State. So people are friendly and we extend that to everybody. It's our way of connecting with people. There are lots of extended families. Hawaiians traditionally take care of everybody. I lived on the mainland*

*for six years and I found that people are not friendly there. Here relationships are
important and it carries into your work. The cornerstone of our healthcare is the
relationship between the member and the physician – that's the most important
thing. Everything else needs to support that relationship. So when we talk about
changes and computerised systems that enable us to do things, we never get away
from that it's the relationship that's the most important thing.*

At first it appeared that Hawaii Kaiser Permanente's institutionalised *aloha, ohana*
and *hanai* were a natural extension of Hawaiian culture. But a more managed
picture emerged. It appeared that, a few years prior to this study, the organisation's culture had been quite dysfunctional and a deliberate effort was made to
transform it by importing some quintessential Hawaiian values. This was successful doubtless because it marked a reassuring return to familiar values held
by Hawaiian employees and members alike.

It also raises an important and wider question concerning the continuity or dis-
continuity of organisations in relation to their cultural context. In the UK, the USA,
and many other countries claiming to be democracies, the behaviour of managers
is often dictatorial. This brand of managerial incompetence has an historical basis
of course, but it means that, for many, the greater part of their lives is conducted
in a context that is quite the opposite of what their society claims to be. In these
circumstances, it would not be surprising if the experience of work were tainted
with dissonance. The managerial prerogative to manage can be synonymous with
a warning above the Company Entrance: 'Democracy Ends Here'.

How refreshing, therefore, to find in Hawaii Kaiser Permanente a nation's
values re-emphasised within the workplace. This cultural continuity was
sufficiently strong in the interviews to be worthy of detailed examination. Let
us first examine how Hawaii Kaiser Permanente culture was consciously
engineered and operationalised. A regional administrator explains:

*Our focus for the last decade has been on caring for Hawaii's people like family.
So this is a mission statement that reflects our vision, and the vision really comes
down to a couple of questions that every doctor might ask themselves: in hiring
a new physician, is this a physician who I will entrust my family members' care
to? (Because we are members of this healthcare insurance format: we get our
care here.) And the second thing is: will I entrust my patients to this physician's
care?*

So Hawaii Kaiser Permanente culture is modelled on an extended family,
including both employees and members. This is seen to be efficient not only to
compete for members but also for staff too:

*'All of the staff are also treated as family. Kaiser Permanente's aim is to be the
employer of choice in healthcare.'*

In fact the primary focus was purportedly on the staff, with members coming
second, because the aim was to cultivate an institution in which members felt
'at home', as another senior administrator explained:

*What we do is create an environment for our staff and our physicians so that they
will feel good about providing service to the members. If people are not happy in
their jobs then we try to put them in the right fit – as long as they are competent.
Because, if people feel good about what they do and their jobs, the rest of it you*

don't have to worry about, because they will do a good job. Then all the other things will come about.

Several other respondents invoked differences between Hawaiian and mainland Kaiser Permanente culture. One implementation team member interpreted the national Kaiser Permanente culture as dominated by its Northern California region. Hawaii Kaiser Permanente was distinctly different from that:

In my opinion Kaiser Permanente Northern California is a very top-down driven organisation. Programs are developed at the top and the thing is, 'You shall do them!' There isn't a whole lot of input coming from the bottom to say, 'Should we really do this, or not?' Here in Hawaii they make a very big push to let everything be controlled at the lowest level possible, and to get a lot of input, a lot of buy-in, a lot of decision making at the lower levels.

The same informant conflated northern California Kaiser Permanente with a ruthless drive for efficiency antithetical to Hawaii Kaiser Permanente:

If you're trying to push automation and efficiency above all else then I think the Northern California approach works well. If you're trying to push the more intimate, one-on-one relationship, then the Hawaii one works. It's not quite as efficient time- and money-wise, but value-wise – I think that's the question. Do the members want a quick service, like calling up Hertz – you don't care who you get, you just want a doctor – or do you want to call up and talk to your personal physician?

He saw the differences between the two regions epitomised in the Hawaii region's fidelity to its core principle: the physician–member relationship. It didn't seem to be the usual managerial rhetoric – rules to espouse and break whenever expedient. The 'core principle' was actually a solid foundation for decision making:

And that's one of the things we push here, and I'm sure you've heard it: our core principle is that the physician–member relationship is the number one thing. At no time do we ever compromise the core principle.

Some informants observed significant differences between Kaiser Permanente regional cultures. They spoke from experience about how those differences mediated organisational innovation, including CIS. Arguably a failure to recognise the culturally mediated nature of implementation is one of the glaring gaps in our understanding of IT innovation and diffusion.

Clinic cultures

A working hypothesis of this study was that an organisation's culture mediates between policy and practice; between what is planned at higher levels of an organisation and what actually happens at a local level. It was predicted that each Hawaiian clinic would exhibit a unique culture and style of leadership – and that the region's culture would be more heterogeneous than the casual observer might expect. These factors would play a part in how CIS was implemented in Hawaii. One Chief was very clear that this was indeed the case:

> *I think there are different cultures in different regions; but there are also different cultures in different clinics. Here, there's a group of 15 internists and their practice culture is very different from the group of 20 internists at [one clinic], and that's very different from a peripheral clinic that is a mixed family practice medicine/paeds, with maybe 10 people in a clinic. The pace of the clinic is different, familiarity with staff is different, expectations of patients for wait times and how busy the wait will be at pharmacy, how long the line will be at X-ray or lab – it's all very different. So inter-regional and intra-regional cultures are different. One size doesn't fit all.*

Another physician working at a clinic remote from the administrative hub of Honolulu noted how its experience of CIS implementation had differed from the more contentious (by Hawaiian standards) experience at other sites:

> *The culture is almost like a kind of troops in the field. We're a little bit away from the centre, so the attitudes can be shaped a little bit easier. Because of that isolation we take a lot of the attitudes from the leadership in the clinic. The acceptance of CIS was pretty much: 'CIS is here, let's deal with it,' as opposed to really challenging [the implementation], 'Should it be here in the first place?' as have some other clinics.*

The same physician added that the active involvement of members of his clinic in the regional implementation process probably influenced their collective experience and evaluation of CIS:

> *Our experience is perhaps a little different in the sense that we had members [...] who really played an integral part in the CIS [implementation]. So we were getting almost weekly updates from these individuals. So it almost became: yes, it was mandated from up high, but our interface was with people that we know, we respected, that we worked with every day, so it was a little bit easier for that message to be accepted.*

Specialty subcultures

It has been argued, not unreasonably, that different medical and surgical specialties would generate distinct subcultures.[64] The medical convention of dividing the body into semi-autonomous physical systems might lead one to expect such an effect. Perhaps this convention has softened slightly over recent years, an effect supported by workflow analysis and team consultations. Even so, most respondents referred to the challenges and opportunities posed *to* implementing CIS *by* different specialties. Some informants emphasised differences between primary and secondary care. For instance, one Chief related how some types of specialty care, including general surgery and obstetrics and gynaecology, were more amenable to computerisation than were other specialties:

> *As we get into CIS, the distinction between primary care and specialty care becomes important. Specialty care is very problem-oriented. You get presented with a problem and you need to fix it. Once it's fixed, barring ongoing complications or problems, then it's done. And then you go to the next patient and you take care of it and it's done. And we lump populations into similar problems. So it's: presented with a problem, fix the problem, end of story. So you can develop algorithms for specific*

problems, like breast problems: how to take care of it, how to approach it, and there's a defined endpoint. And that sometimes lends itself to computerisation.

The same Chief argued that a similar translation into algorithms would be impossible for primary care, at least with CIS:

You get into primary care and the complaint can come in all over the map, you know, and you can't write an algorithm for primary care. And then it becomes a problem of one-on-one discussion and feeling it out in terms of how you solve their problem – or how you manage it actually. You don't really solve their problems: you just sort of manage them over the life of the patient. You basically go with them for their lifetime and you manage their health problems, as it relates to whatever – in their lives, or in their social lives, professional lives, or whatever, or their physical life, or spiritual life. There's no specific to it.

Thus he characterised primary care as offering a lifetime of medical and social support, whereas certain specialties offered discrete interventions and set pieces:

You have a set problem that we have to fix. The history that you have to take is pretty well known. The physical examination you know what to expect. And the studies that you'd need to support or refute those diagnoses are pretty much known, so you already have them set up in the CIS system. So it can be structured pretty nicely actually – and the procedures. So because of that algorithmic style you can actually structure it in a computer. So there's less ambiguity. When you pull up your diagnoses, you don't have to go hunting for something weird that often. Whereas in primary care: oh man, you don't know what's going to walk through the door.

Supporting that view, another Chief noted a stronger individualism among surgeons compared with other specialties:

Paediatricians and family practitioners tend to be a little more, 'Let's all get together; let's go forward as a group; let's play together'. Surgeons tend to be a lot more independent; a lot more entrepreneurial, but not in the financial sense: in an independence and practice sense. And the 'herding cats' analogy is certainly an apt one, or someone else said 'herding bumblebees'. Basically, just by saying that we should all do this, you create poles of people saying, 'Well, if you say that, obviously we should think about it and maybe not *do it'.*

We note in passing how paradoxical this resistance to organisation is inasmuch as it denotes an *institutionalised* individualism defined (collectively) via membership of a specialty. Surgeons' awareness and avowal of their individualistic tendency was probably enhanced by its eccentricity in relation to the collectivist beliefs underpinning Hawaiian culture and the Asian cultures to which many Kaiser Permanente physicians also belonged.

Of course some specialties, including internal medicine and OB/GYN, deliver primary and secondary care. That prompted them to consider whether all or which parts of their practice were amenable to computerisation, as another Chief related:

We are not as individualistic as general surgery. And then we do primary care too, which is OB and day-to-day gynaecology, which is almost more primary care than it is specialty care, everything from routine exams to vaginal infections and other acute care. So we're kind of a mix between primary care and surgical care.

It is generally assumed that the electronic medical record is pivotal to quality improvement. A physician can be more reliably informed of a patient's most recent history than with hard copy records. That was confirmed by many respondents, though one Chief thought it less of an advantage to certain specialties than to others. In his own practice:

> *Patients usually come in for a problem that they are familiar with. They walk in and say, 'Doc, I'm here because of X'. I don't need to go to a chart note to find that out. Yeh, I can go and look at some of the history, but I'm going to retake that anyway. It really wasn't very useful to me to go to that note unless the patient came in and said, 'Doc, I've no idea why I'm here.'*

It might be predicted that the implementation of CIS would tend to converge disparate practice patterns – among independent-minded surgeons, for instance. This point was generally conceded by respondents – but within limits, as one Chief explained:

> *A team approach means relinquishing a little bit of autonomy but mostly it's about changing one's style of doing medicine. Style has a lot to do with medicine – personal style, how you approach people and problems.*
>
> *There is reasonable standardisation of process, but surgeons tend to be fiercely individualistic, so that is the culture of the department. And the reason it becomes that way, and I think it's quite similar for doctors and specifically gynaecologists, is that it's a one-on-one delivery of care. If it goes well you get rewarded; and if it goes badly you, you know, get hurt by it. And that's why it's fiercely individualistic: when things go right or wrong, other people are not getting patted on the back or hit on the head – it's you. So that's the whole character and flavour of the practice. You can't really tell people what to do because you're not next to them when things go wrong.*

Another Chief qualified the point by noting the context dependency of modes of practice even within the same specialty. Thus, care delivered by equivalent clinicians would inevitably differ according to their location and the mix of expertise available:

> *We do things 20 different ways, or however many people we have. But we're organised differently. For example, General Surgery is all here, on one location, whereas we have four locations on Oahu. Then we have a growing group of nine on Maui. So we create teams in the separate locations. In [another clinic] there are six and there are three and two in other locations. So from that perspective there's a different team approach, which means different ways of working together.*

Cultures and implementation

Some respondents described Hawaii Kaiser Permanente culture in terms of a distribution of personality types. One member of the implementation team referred to a psychological typing exercise, apparently undertaken prior to implementing CIS, and how this had helped him to make sense of responses to innovation:

We've done these profile studies, and I forget what you call them, but there is the Amiable group, the Driver group, Expressives and then the Analytics. We've all been given this test to show what categories we are in so that we can tell it to each other: 'Well you're an Amiable and therefore you feel this way, and I'm an Analytic.' Basically we are 70% Amiable! There's a little bit of unbalance there:

'You wanna do which? OK we can do that – how soon do you want it?'
'Is there any problem here?'
'No, everything is fine!'

Here, apparently, we find the Western analytical gaze refracted by a benign Hawaiian duplicity. What to systems engineers and cyberneticists appears as corrective negative feedback leading to systematic error reduction, is by amiable Hawaiians seen to impugn personal integrity, leading to conflict and alienation. Both are right in their own terms and wrong in each other's. The same CIS team member outlined the implications of this culture clash for evaluating implementation:

It's hard getting real constructive criticism out of people because we have such a strong drive for team building and doing things together that to be the dissident voice is almost seen to be unpatriotic. A lot of Amiables find it hard to say: 'Wait a minute – I don't think this is going to work'.

It's very important that we get along: everybody knows that. You want to be seen to be getting along. We spend so much time in team building that if you're not a team player, it's not good. It's the natural culture of Hawaii to be very polite. We don't beep our horn; we don't cut our way in line. You never talk stink. That's a phrase that's used here: 'You don't talk stink.' You don't say bad things about other people. If you give constructive feedback, if somebody asks for it, they are in a little bit of a shock if they actually get it. So culture: big influence here.

Another implementation team member described Kaiser Permanente culture as a complex weave of clinical and administrative threads, reflecting Kaiser Permanente's dual structure: Kaiser Health Plan and Permanente Medical Groups operating hand in glove, providing prepaid health insurance on the one side, and health services on the other:

And the culture is twofold. In our organisation we have a business or clinical leadership culture, and we have a medical culture, and there's two leaders who partner at each level. So you have potentially two threads of culture running through the same building. At a large clinic you've got a physician lead, and you've got an Area Manager. That Area Manager might run the nursing supervisors in a very positive way, but that physician just may cut that process off at the knees because they are more of a lone ranger in the way that they like to do things. And so we tend to do a lot of work with our Area Managers trying to bring our chiefs along.

Finally, under the culture heading, one clinic Chief reported having deliberately worked to improve a dysfunctional clinic culture, underlining earlier observations concerning the heterogeneity of Hawaii Kaiser Permanente, and how unsafe it was to conceive each location merely as a fragment of a homogeneous organisation or organisational culture. In contrast to such a corporate image, each site was presented as a unique, complex, dynamic subsystem of healthcare administration and delivery; clinics differing in detail as well as sharing common characteristics.

Hence, although guided by a common ethos, Hawaii Kaiser Permanente culture was a distributed and heterogeneous phenomenon that could only be located across all its sites:

> When I became Chief the clinic was having a lot of morale problems, problems working as a team. Everybody was kinda out for themselves. You know, like 'I'm not gonna help anybody, I'm just gonna try and get through the day myself'. I think we tried to change that into: 'We are gonna help each other, and we're gonna all get through it together.' Instead of one person staying till nine o'clock, maybe if we all pitched in we could all get out together.

Implicit in this Chief's account is a narrative of survival rather than success or effectiveness. The question it implies is not 'How can we excel at implementing CIS?' but rather 'How can we strengthen our clinical culture to help withstand the impact of implementing CIS?' The former implies a radical, the latter a conservative impulse. We do not mean that this clinic intended to react against CIS, but that its first priority was to organise the conditions of its own survival, inextricably linked to the provision of services to its members.

Leadership

The medical leadership was represented as democratic, consultative and consensus-seeking, at least from the perspective of physicians, as one CIS trainer explained:

> One thing coming down from our senior leader: we very rarely mandate anything. His thinking is that if it's a good thing it'll get a critical mass and it will take hold. And if it's not a good thing then it won't. So, as we roll it out to the various clinics, I think he won't tell his chiefs that anything has to be done relative to our project. He firmly believes in the electronic health record. It's a very difficult road to go down; it's a very expensive road to go down. And I think politically it's a ship he doesn't want to sail on unless it gets buy-in.

Another implementation team member noted that:

> It was a very noticeable difference between Colorado region and Hawaii: a very different culture. It's very collaborative, very consensus-driven, a sense of...the Hawaiian word is ohana, the family. Part of that is probably driven by the high percentage of Asian culture that we have here. They really don't want to be in conflict with people, it's not their style to be very pedantic about things. From a management style people don't want to walk up to you and say, 'Thou shalt do this.' They'd rather come up and say, 'Wouldn't it be a really good idea if we did this?' Just wanting to get a lot of buy-in, a lot of consensus. It's been very successful for the region. They've spent quite a lot of money and time educating folks to instil that kind of thinking.

That style of leadership harmonised with Hawaiian culture, but was not seen to be very conducive to CIS implementation. Several implementation team members thought the search for consensus slowed the pace of implementation, yet also led to a better outcome overall:

There are also some downsides. Because we try to get a whole lot of input we typically have a longer implementation period. By trying to get the momentum going before we put it out there. I think that's right because if you spend more time up front, you spend less time cleaning up at the back end.

The high value placed on achieving consensus and maintaining relationships meant that decision making could be notoriously slow. Some respondents expressed bemusement and frustration at this but accepted it as an inevitable part of Hawaiian, and Hawaii Kaiser Permanente, culture. In addition, administrators acknowledged that physicians were influenced mainly by their professional colleagues, but also that professional courtesy proscribed coercive methods of persuasion between physicians. Thus the approach to CIS implementation appeared to depend on a power of demonstration by reference group. If CIS were a good system it would stand the test of initial implementation by clinicians of acknowledged competence and credibility. That was a deliberate strategy. But some informants perceived a strong ambiguity in the stance of leaders, who may have harboured private misgivings about CIS but nonetheless felt duty bound to promote its implementation:

You know everybody says – and indeed I think its true – [that] to get this kind of quantum change in how people work – it's a huge change, having to do it electronically, you need very strong sponsorship. So I think in all fairness, our top-level sponsors: they were struggling with, 'This is a turkey and I gotta make people...' So he waxed and waned and he was in a very, very difficult position to deal with that. And so on down into the higher management levels. Everybody had a real struggle. They knew they had to do a good job as sponsors, and yet you're trying to defend something you don't really believe in.

Though some informants were mildly critical, none expressed a desire to change the leadership style, or the culture in which it was embedded. According to a senior administrator:

There's something that's been pretty important about our culture. We eschew authoritarian leadership. We don't think it works. We believe that a more important function of leadership is having the right people doing the right work and getting the feedback that you need as a leader to remove barriers.

The same informant conceded that such a permissive style of leadership might appear less effective than a more authoritarian approach – not to Hawaii Kaiser Permanente employees, but to the national organisation:

We have our failings. If we had been more authoritative at certain times, I don't think it would have improved our implementation. But it would have improved our understanding with the national organisation, and their priorities and what their promise was to us. So it's not always flowers and love [reference to aloha].

One Chief was more explicitly critical of Kaiser Permanente national HQ:

Program Office even criticised our leaders for showing bad leadership because they were not supporting their line, you know, 'CIS will work, CIS will work.' Even our leaders started saying, 'There's better stuff out there.'

The same Chief referred to the dilemma in which Hawaii Kaiser Permanente found itself: committed to implementing a system it knew to be seriously flawed:

In the beginning, they did pound it home: the project team leaders were as militant supporters of CIS as anyone. But then they saw what was happening. It was too clumsy, and they didn't take enough time to get buy-in from docs. They didn't take into account local culture. It got to where Program Office was ignoring the project team leaders, who still very obediently tried their best with their hands tied. And I think people in the front line started seeing that they are not the masterminds of evil here: they are the messengers. We shouldn't be throwing rocks at them. I saw that change at about nine months.

The same respondent interpreted the new Kaiser Permanente Chief Executive's decision to abort the implementation of CIS as vindication of the local leadership:

When [the new senior leaders] came that really restored faith – that, 'Wow, somebody really is listening and they are willing to take a step back.' Leadership resurrected the positive momentum we have now toward Epic. That didn't come locally, I think that came from [the new senior leaders]. It took the leadership change at the highest levels to do that.

Criticism of Kaiser Permanente national leadership prior to the changes at the top were articulated in literally vocal terms by an implementation team member:

Over here the small voice can be heard. I believe I've had a lot of personal impact on the organisation, whereas in Northern California you really are lost. Here the small voice has access to the leadership. It's a very caring leadership, they listen to us; they even get emotional with us. I think as much as possible they are very frank with their thinking and where the organisation is going.

The same person was, however, careful to note differences in Hawaii leadership styles:

There's a Chief at one clinic whose attitude was: implementing CIS was like us taking the beach at Normandy: we're gonna do it. Then there were others who were more, 'Well, let's think about this' and 'do we really want this? And I want to hear everybody's opinion.' So there was both. I would say more Chiefs would be inclined to be of the Amiable type and quietly say, 'Well if that is where everybody is going and that is what we need to do, we just need to fall in line and show our support for it.'

The Chief does carry a lot of weight here. We don't go anywhere and make any operational decisions unless the physicians and specifically the Chiefs are involved and give it their OK. And we look to them to set the example and the standard and then when necessary to get up and speak to the group and give the motivational speech.

A dilemma between public commitment and private doubt regarding CIS apparently spread throughout the organisation. A strong desire to conform to institutional expectations conflicted with a strong desire to maintain high professional standards and efficiency. Participants were in a dilemma between apprehending CIS as a system presented to doctors as something that they needed to comply with, and as something that they could make use of for their practice: something for them, not something that they had to oblige the organisation by taking on board:

That is a critical difference. So there was that tug-of-war going on. Yes, the leadership did everything they could to empower the physicians. It was very difficult. Leadership used all the right words. They also wanted to implement it. And therefore a timetable was set which was very aggressive. And they [the physicians] all looked at that timetable and said, 'Well, we have no choice but to go along!' So I think they saw mixed signals. They felt mixed signals I should say. There was the signal, 'We've got to implement this' and there is themselves saying, 'Well we've got to make it work for us, and if I don't feel comfortable with it, then what should I do?' And it was very hard for physicians to speak out.

This dilemma and the mixed signals received from leaders made the task of implementing CIS still harder. That in turn led implementation team members to realise the importance of strong leadership in such circumstances, as the following passage attests:

The ease or difficulty with which CIS can be implemented depends on the leadership, primarily the physician leadership. If the physician leadership is strong and willing to change their way of practice – and willing to hold their people accountable to doing the change, as well as themselves, which is critical, we have an easier time. I don't think it's an easier time for the individual physician, but for us it's easier to work with those groups. And I think in the long term it's those groups that have been most successful.

If the leadership is very wary, then usually they end up either not going, or going – but then you find pieces of their departments falling backwards. And it's harder to support, because [in] an area that's committed to going in one direction, we can help the folks that have difficulty because there is commitment to the change. As the commitment dwindles it's much harder to get them to where they want to be, as a group.

Another team member endorsed that view:

We've learned that sponsorship and leadership are the most important aspects of the deployment: because without the sponsorship of the areas; without our team leaders working with the Chiefs, we really had no authority in going in to do any kind of process improvement without their support. And it's an infrastructure that will hold for Epic.

Another respondent specified the kinds of leadership behaviour required for successful implementation, and perhaps unwittingly offered an alternative and complementary derivation of the initials EMR:

Express, model and reinforce. If we do that as a group we'll be much more successful. Express what you want, model it – do it – and reinforce it. And if we can do those three things all the way up and down the chain, we'll be successful. The leadership need to say it, model it and reinforce it. We can support that because then every person should be doing the same thing. It really is more about people than it is about technology.

But the social dimension of leadership could not be separated from the technical characteristics of the system. Perceiving ambiguity among leaders about the desirability of implementing CIS in their practices, it would be natural for physicians to then consider the consequences of not complying. This became a substantial concern to the implementation team. If non-compliance was not penalised, then economy of effort alone could be a sufficient barrier to adoption by individual clinics and physicians, and any technical considerations could be used to rationalise inertia. As one team member noted, ambivalence at the top combined with a low risk of censure permitted – even encouraged – non-participation:

> *There has been some hesitance with CIS at the very highest levels of our organisation. I don't think the physician Chiefs or individuals who have not fulfilled their CIS commitment feel any repercussions. In fact they have been told 'It's OK'. So they don't really have anything to worry about by saying 'No'.*
>
> *From a change management perspective that was the nightmare, because we depended on the Chiefs and the supervisors of the clinic to be really clear about what their expectations were in terms of performance in CIS.*
>
> *It was hard for them to delineate the positive and negative consequences related to those performance expectations. As part of change management, consequences are real critical to changing behaviour. Setting the expectations was a challenge: having them verbalise and commit to positive and negative consequences for that performance was even more of a challenge. […] We had to coach a lot of the leadership in, 'What are your expectations? How are you gonna to verbalise it? When are you going to verbalise it? In what meeting; what's the agenda?' So we did a lot of behind-the-scenes prepping for the leadership to manage the transition, even after we leave.*

This was doubly significant, as it appeared to have left a lingering doubt about the success of the impending implementation of Epic:

> *So it will be interesting to see what will happen, because Epic is more accepted by the leadership, who see it as something that the physicians can do more easily and won't be as stressful to them. So hopefully, if the same issues come up, with, 'Well I don't care if it's CIS or Epic, I'm not going to play!' then there will be more pressure on them to conform – but I'll believe it when I see it.*

That scepticism was partly explained by the uneven state of readiness to implement encountered in the region, and whether senior leaders had acquired the ability to deal with laggards effectively, as another member of the team noted:

> *There are some people that, despite the fact that the product has a lot of problems, like it, use it and wouldn't want to go back to paper. On the other hand we had a whole bunch of departments that were contesting to go up last; and there were people who weren't going to do it no matter what you did to them!*

As with any healthcare innovation, the fate of CIS was bound up with the status of Permanente physicians as independent professionals who, despite being mainly salaried, nonetheless hold at least partial allegiance to institutions transcending any specific healthcare provider organisation: the institution of medicine itself. Not so for nursing. Owing to a spirit of independence (Saint Simon, one of the founding fathers of sociology, termed it 'cosmopolitanism') born of professional, trans-organisational solidarity, there was little felt need for physicians to dissemble about their personal intentions to implement or not to implement CIS, as this implementation team member noted:

> *I don't think any of the clinics set out to mislead us about their level of commitment.*

I think the chiefs knew – and we know – who we were going to have problems with – and they were open about it. Now, who was going to deal with those problems was always the question. We could help with more training, more support, more one-on-one work; but other than that there's always been the question – even from the chiefs themselves. 'Now, after all that, if I still got somebody who can't do it, or won't play, what kind of support will I get from the very highest levels of the physician organisation to deal with this?' And I don't know that they ever really got an answer for that. Whereas with nursing supervisors it's like, 'Do it, or else.' You know if you don't do it you're out of a job.

These very practical considerations required CIS trainers to coach physician leaders in handling dissent and disagreement among those who, for administrative purposes, were their 'staff' – but were also their professional peers.

As one implementation team member described, coaching leaders to manage dissent among physicians in ways that would minimise the risk of breaching professional etiquette; or among non-physicians (nurses, medical assistants, therapists) in ways more sensitive than apparent brutal indifference, posed yet another challenge:

A lot of change management is preparing leaders for staff reactions, teaching them, 'These are the things you have to be ready to respond to. What are the words you are going to say, how are you going to deal with that? Because people are going to respond to this change negatively and positively. It's not about you: it's about them and what's happening in their lives and in their world. How are you going to respond to that?'

When I was a Chief those are the kind of skills no one ever talked to me about, but they are very helpful skills for a lot of projects that you do, a lot of changes that you make.

One CIS team member remarked that some physicians with formal leadership roles actually exhibited little if any discernible leadership behaviour:

And some of the people who were in leadership roles or sponsorship roles were not really doing much active leading or sponsoring. And that's just typical of an organisation where some people are just floating along.

Another team member noted that physicians were generally unused to active leadership and tended only to intervene in exceptional situations:

I think the Chiefs often only deal with outside the 95th percentile of behaviour: rewarding the people who are doing great and working on the major problems; and dealing with patient complaints and that kind of stuff. In our organisation the medical culture is pretty forgiving, consensus-driven. Mandates don't come down from above – which drives some people crazy because like, 'Are we gonna all do this?' We know we are all gonna do it but nobody is going to come up and say, 'You have to do it now and if you don't you should start looking for another job.' It's very permissive.

It seemed that nurse supervisors and clinic managers did most of the local shaking and moving, with the physician Chief weighing in only when a situation fell outside their authority. The same respondent explained how this had worked and how CIS implementation had induced some physicians to take a more active leadership role:

> *Generally, there are physician leaders and then there are their supervisor partners and then clinic managers. The clinic managers generally have the more solid sponsorship roles, and then the supervisors next; and then the Chiefs often are just putting out fires or trying to keep the status quo.*

So, how did this patchwork of leadership and clinic readiness affect CIS implementation? One Chief related clinics' responses to their attitudes to change. But he also implied that a Chief who exhibited strong sponsorship of CIS could in practice overcome negative attitudes:

> *I think a lot of the differences between the teams and between the clinics, in terms of why some were easier than others, had to do with a whole attitude of change. That was the biggest factor. If your leaders weren't really for it that was crucial. Internal medicine at [one clinic] never did go up. They haven't even used partial functionality. It was the leadership in that department that this was not the system.*

One specialty with strong leadership was induced to go onto the system regardless of individual attitudes, however, as a clinic manager noted:

> *In OB/GYN the leadership was terrific, so implementing OB here and at [this clinic] went very well. It was more autocratic. A decision was made – 'That is how it is going be' – so that made it easier for the team to roll it out. Because it was real clear for the team, really clear.*

In addition to that directive approach, however, we should recall that other respondents distinguished between specialties in terms of their amenability to computerisation ('We are simple people doing simple procedures'). So it is realistic to think of leadership as a necessary but not sufficient factor in the equation of readiness to implement CIS: leadership as one cultural or ecological factor. Another factor was the capacity or intensity of a clinic's or department's work. If clinicians felt overburdened, perhaps only a visionary leader could have inspired them to change their practices and endure the extra burden of implementing – and using – CIS, as another clinic manager noted:

> *I think the physician leadership at the time of the implementation was not as strong as it could be. For instance, when we asked, 'What is the outcome that you hope to achieve when we're done with this, what would success look like to you?' success was defined as 'getting through my day'. It's really hard to get people excited about getting through their day. Whereas another clinic could define it as, 'having information at my fingertips and being on the cutting edge of technology in medicine' and all the benefits that would accrue.*

Ultimately, regional leaders were vindicated. They learned from CIS that any electronic medical record system was likely to exacerbate the access challenges they already faced. They concluded from this that an even more radical transformation of the healthcare model would be necessary, as one Chief said:

> *I have to respect the leadership: I think they see that the folk in the trenches are working really hard, and we need to change the system for us to survive. In that sense, I really don't think CIS was a failure because it made us rethink things.*

Hence, there is a need to revise not only judgements of success and failure as such, but the adequacy of success and failure as evaluative criteria. Which is another way of distinguishing between single-loop and double-loop feedback.[3] In particular, there is a need to view evaluation formatively and diachronically, and to play down the summative, synchronic finality of judgement. The implementation of CIS suggests that a failed implementation may become a learning platform and equip an organisation for future success. As long as success and failure are exploited as learning, perhaps no intervention wholly fails. Conversely, the most resounding success may lead to future failure if it blunts the spur to continuous improvement through innovation.

Whether these statements appear trite, or post-hoc rationalisations, probably depends on one's perspective or paradigm. Our encounters with the implementation team discovered a learning ethos in which implementation was viewed as an iterative, recursive task, rather than a unique intervention. In addition, all the team members we interviewed were Hawaii Kaiser Permanente employees. For them the researcher/consultant's adage about getting in, getting on, and getting out did *not* apply. The operative ethos was getting on and *continuing* to get on with colleagues in the long run. Like leadership, therefore, success and failure are slippery concepts.[70] Revising such abstract concepts is an important part of restoring technological innovation to its social organisational context.

The approach to implementation

The choice of the initial implementation sites was guided by an awareness of diffusion theory combined with a detailed knowledge of clinic cultures and individual personalities. The first site to go up was a small clinic of four physicians, the clinic Chief being a keen supporter of computerisation. Although often termed a pilot site its role relative to the implementation of CIS was ambiguous. It was unclear, for instance, whether the CIS rollout was contingent on successful implementation at the first clinic. One informant reported that there *were* stopping rules, but that aborting the rollout was never seriously considered – until it became known that Kaiser Permanente was reviewing its options nationally. CIS had been fully implemented in one third of clinics in Kaiser Permanente, though even 'full' implementation did not necessarily mean that everyone at a site was using all its functions. Almost all other clinics had read-only access, of which some also had the order entry function. However, the precise utilisation of CIS in clinics is not really known. It was reported that even fully implemented clinics reverted to paper at times, and at least one specialty clinic with read-only access hardly used CIS at all, if ever.

The devil, as usual, is in the detail. To state that CIS had or had not been implemented in a given site may tell as much about a system of classification as what actually happened. And even statements such as '100% implementation' at a given site cannot be relied upon to mean what they seem. We must recognise that the actual implementation of CIS in Hawaii and any account of that implementation are two different things: one lived through, the other a narrative. But sometimes one gets a deeper insight into the one through the other. An example of this was when a clinic manager mentioned that OB/GYN, which almost all other respondents had exemplified as being 100% on CIS, was not in fact quite so:

> *The leadership also identified areas where the electronic medical record was weak and where it wouldn't support their efforts well. I think that contributed to their success, because they used the system where it was strong and it supported their practice, and they chose not to use it where it would be problematic. So they used the system in their 80%, which is their gynaecological patients, and didn't use it in their obstetrics patients, where it was problematic; it could create various workflow problems, documentation problems or provider problems, and so they kept that out of the system and continued to document in the paper way.*

When it was stated that OB/GYN was up on CIS 100%, that is not a literal description, but a classification. This alerts us to the probability that other clinics and specialties may have actively discriminated between those parts of their work that were more or less amenable to computerisation with CIS.

Respondents emphasised that Hawaii had volunteered as the first region to implement the new version of CIS (an earlier version having been used in Colorado region for several years), as this regional administrator states:

> *Hawaii volunteered to go first, our choice entirely. We said we want to be at the front of the line. We have the culture, the cooperation within the group. We understand the need for an electronic health record. We want the clinical advantages. But we think that our readiness to change is at a high enough level that we will be successful, and that you can model what we do here.*

That enthusiasm was informed by a cogent change management strategy. Behind the laissez-faire public face of regional management there were hints that perhaps the region's culture was being engineered by one or two directing minds, as the philosophy espoused by another regional administrator implies:

> *We in Hawaii have gone through so many changes. We have lots of competition out there, so we have to be good in what we do. We've had major changes: development of teams…And because we concentrate on people we make sure that all the principles of change management are addressed. Which means that we always get people ready; we make sure they understand the big 'Why?' Why they are doing things. People that work with us have a high degree of commitment. So they are ready, they want to make the organisation better, so they are willing to make changes. So we are ready for change – there is a readiness for change. The way that we do it is, you work with the early adopters, and then you get more and more people on board and before you know it everybody is on board.*

A training team member also used the lexicon of innovation diffusion to discuss differences in readiness and ability to implement within and between sites:

> *I really have a learner's approach to things. So I expect a heterogeneous community whenever I go into a new training endeavour, a bell-shaped curve. You'll have your early adopters; the mass group that's kind of, 'Well, we'll do it because we've been told to'; and then you'll have the people that are hyper-resistant at the other end of the bell curve – for multiple reasons. I've always valued that diversity because the trainers and support specialists can't do everybody at the same time. So from a scheduling perspective it has helped us.*

> *Using the early adopters is a bit like catching a wave: you can shoot forward a bit; use their energy quite a bit. Actually that's one of our strategies – to get more and more people on board besides the project team.*

This approach draws on innovation diffusion theory.[64] One insight is that diffusion can occur only if an innovation can be translated into the organisation's culture.* As we have seen, the voluntarism favoured by Hawaii Kaiser Permanente's leaders set the tone for its approach to strategic change management, as one administrator describes:

> *I have to give a lot of credit to our Medical Director: he never forces people to do things. His whole philosophy is, 'People will come on board because already we have committed people.' Some of their commitment is like, 'OK, if it doesn't work we are going to say it doesn't work and we going to pressure you to change it.' That was pervasive also. Some of the departments said, 'We are not going to do this, because we don't think this is the right one,' and they kept pushing that, pushing that. And so he went to bat out there with national, 'This isn't working now for us.'*
>
> *So we put the ones that resisted at the end of the implementation. Because after a while if the masses are saying, 'This is good,' the rest of them will come on board. It just takes time. But we are very good at knowing who will be the first ones to do it and do it well. So it takes a lot of judgement and understanding people and understanding where they are at.*

We have seen that regional leaders had faith in the ability of early adopters to convince the mass of physicians to implement CIS. It was hoped that eventually even the most sceptical would be faced with no alternative than to use CIS. With so much at stake, it made sense to choose a small clinic to go up first, as one respondent explained:

> *My thinking about why they were chosen to be the first clinic has changed over time. Initially, I thought they were chosen because they had a record of achievement, excellent patient satisfaction, quality of care, staff satisfaction. The physicians were also relatively young, reasonably comfortable with the technology and, being small, they could move quickly.*
>
> *My personal feeling about this is that we have to move to an electronic patient record: it's crazy not to make use of this technology and if any clinic was going to be successful at it, it surely would be that clinic, because they've got the all-star team, they've got the right attitude. So if it was coming anyway, why not reap the benefits of being the first? And they might have an opportunity to influence the whole implementation in a positive way.*
>
> *In retrospect I realise that a very good reason to be first was because it was 'expendable' too. If it went up in flames, it's just one small clinic, and we're not taking down the whole organisation, whereas if it was a large clinic, if this failed, that would have a huge impact on the organisation. So it's a cynical view but it makes perfect sense, and it was a smart decision.*

---

*In an early illustrative study of technological innovation, most of a village's women could not be persuaded to boil contaminated water as they lacked any microbial theory of disease – heat sterilisation did not make sense to them. Moreover, it was found that the innovations could only be communicated successfully by respected cultural insiders.

When a CIS team member was asked if a different style of leadership might have increased the success of the implementation, the answer reflected the attitude held by most other respondents: that Hawaii Kaiser Permanente had the kind of leadership that befitted its medical culture:

> *The approach to implementation could have been more authoritative. But it would have been anti-culture; very anti-culture – on the medical group side – not so much on the nursing side. Nurses are used to being ordered about and they're more used to the consequences.*

One respondent compared the Hawaii implementation to the implementation of the earlier version in Colorado region and drew comparisons between their approaches to leading change management:

> *There were certainly efforts to recognise change management in Colorado, but Colorado took a more aggressive approach, got through the training in the region in a much shorter timeframe, just because of the way the organisation works; they were able to chunk people up in a different manner. Works for Colorado, doesn't work in Hawaii – just because of cultural and political differences.*
>
> *The typical doctor–staff hierarchy isn't as prevalent in Kaiser as it may be in other medical organisations. However, the reality of it is: if you don't have buy-in from your medical group, your MDs, in whatever project you're pursuing, your project is probably not going to succeed very far.*

Was the first site a pilot?

As noted, the pilot status of the first clinic was ambiguous and a range of opinions was found regarding what being the pilot site meant. Was it a true pilot site, or simply first in the rollout? A clinic Chief was first to raise this issue:

> *There was also some question about their role. There was the question: 'Is this a pilot?' And the CIS leadership tried to make it clear that they were not a pilot. They specifically said: 'Do not call this a pilot: you are the first clinic or the initial site.'*

So why did some informants think otherwise? Was it just assumed to be a pilot; was there a change of official view; were mixed messages received? A CIS team member:

> *There were differing perceptions about the status of the first clinic implementation, with some seeing it as a pilot and others not. And even among many of the key people on the leadership team, there were some who expressed the opinion that, 'No, we are going ahead'.*
>
> *The first site was supposed to be the testing ground, the 'lab'. And I was told: 'No, this is not a lab: we are implementing this thing.' I thought there should have been more physicians involved in looking at that, to get more input. It was a default decision: 'Well nobody's really disagreeing, so let's move ahead.'*
>
> *I don't think we were all unified in that voice. National left us alone, as far as I know.*

One of the clinic managers was clear, and still maintained, that the first clinic *had* been a pilot:

> *A: And it was a pilot. It was a pilot.*
> *Q: It was a pilot?*
> *A: Yes.*

But another clinic manager was equally sure that it had *not* been a pilot, even though it was called such:

> *Initially everyone referred to the first clinic as a pilot site, but I don't think there was ever any intent to make the rollout contingent on whether it was a success there. It was, 'We are going to implement it at [a small urban clinic], we're going to look and learn from it, and then we're going to roll through the rest of the organisation.' It was called a pilot for quite some time, and then there was some difficulty in changing the nomenclature.*
>
> *There was a lot of confusion among the clinic staff about whether they were a pilot or not. So as we went to implementation we told them, 'You're the initial site.' I think they changed it from pilot site to initial site somewhere really close to implementation. I don't think anybody ever thought, 'If it doesn't work there, we're just going stop and say "we don't want to do this any more".'*

Perhaps the confusion was due to loose terminology. But it was a significant issue to participants at the first site. If it were a true pilot, an $800 million investment might have appeared to depend upon their actions. If they were merely the initial site they would be under much less pressure. As a pilot, the clinic was also being tested; as initial site, CIS was being tested at that site among others. It's potentially a big difference. It would be facile to recommend more clarity concerning pilot sites, but more valuable to pick up on the fact that, amid all the preparatory and design work, it is quite likely that clarity will be absent concerning some key issues running up to implementation. Implementation is of necessity a formative process and sometimes it may be wiser not to try to specify every aspect too precisely.

Workflow analysis

How, then, did the CIS team prepare the ground for implementation? They did not simply show up with the software. A great deal of pre-implementation work was undertaken, particularly at the first clinic. The extent of preparation at that site was part planned, part contingent, as the 14-month delay in delivery had created an activity vacuum to be filled. Here and at other clinics an internal team of organisational engineers went in to analyse systems and workflows, as one administrator described:

> *Organisational engineers walked through the system asking, 'How do you check patients in? Where do they go next?' So understanding workflows within the clinic settings, which were found to be quite different across locations, depending on the size of the clinic and the clientele.*

We have noted that CIS was implemented within a context of ongoing quality improvement initiatives. One care process redesign initiative was termed *patient flow improvement*: a clinic manager explained:

We started our patient flow improvement process in 1999. And then we were preparing to come up in 2000 and didn't actually come up until 2001. We began [by mapping] how the patient moves through our clinic – from a patient's point of view, and trying to identify all of those points along the line, and then identify the steps, and looking for redundancy or inefficiency or clarity, understanding, so the patient had a better experience with us.

According to one clinic manager, the patient flow improvement process actually pre-dated CIS. It was followed by another 'patient flow straw man process'. This altered the analysis from the movement of patients through a clinic to the care processes which they encountered there. The following excerpt suggests how communication boundaries and insular individual practices began to be broken down:

Then we did what we called our 'patient flow straw man process'. We would put up a straw man of every clinic process, and then we would have a team meeting for the physicians, appointment clerks, nurse: everybody got in a room and said 'OK: is this how it goes?' And the receptionist goes, 'I don't do that – this is what I do.' And the doctor would go, 'Well, why do you do that?' Or, 'If you do that I don't need to do that.' Or the RNs would say, 'Well I'm doing this.' And the physicians go, 'Well, why are you doing that? The MAs can do that.' So it was really a good dialogue and process.

Whether or not those improvements were planned as part of CIS, their potential to support the implementation program quickly became evident to those involved:

We started this process at one clinic and we said, 'Wow! We should use this tool as we implement CIS.' So, when CIS was coming, we stepped it up a notch. So it's, 'OK, now we have this other "person"' – we called it the Cisco Kid – 'in the exam room with you and how do you integrate CIS into the equation?' So we then took this patient flow straw man process and did the same thing using CIS.

But the process improvement team went further than inducing clinicians to *describe* their working habits to one another; they proceeded to introduce peer assessment, as the same clinic manager reported:

Then we had the doctors actually view each other as they worked with a patient, and they gained new knowledge from each other on efficiencies, shortcuts and their practice styles.

At the same time we tried to bring the staff up to a competency level of support, of getting things ready for the physician. This helped a lot because then we could figure out what we could take off some of their plates; what kinds of things we needed to improve on. And we had a big bulletin board where we had each one of these processes: registration, workup, discharge; and then as we changed things we would put that up there.

Striking in these passages is the revelatory tone in which new ways of sharing information about individual practices are discussed. It implies that each person's practice was by default their own business – not literally, in this mainly salaried context, but that each clinician was their own master or mistress. It is hard to see how with that ethos quality could reliably have been assured. The lack of previous standardisation and team process suggests that physicians were idiosyncratic, each practising personal variations on standard medical techniques. This not only contained a worrying implication of obscurity (by which we mean working in the semi-darkness of one's own insular and potentially eccentric practice) but that practitioners might be forced by convention to struggle alone to master techniques and approaches to medical problems that a little more communication with their fellow practitioners might facilitate.

Kaiser Permanente's prepaid group practice ethos has fostered many advantages over solo practice since 1937. Indeed, as we see below, team building in Hawaii region began several years prior to CIS. Yet there was still a strong sense in which, even in group practices, the fundamental individualism of medical practitioners reigned. Sharing information about their practices seemed to have been an epiphany for some physicians, and nurses. As one CIS team member noted, however, the physician's prerogative to practise in his or her own distinctive way was actually supported by the implementation's ethos:

> One of our principles is that doctors need to be able to practise in a style that works for them. And so we worked hard to discover ways, workflows, different ways of clicking, different ways of working from an exam room to a nursing station, to help them find their stride. And there just seemed to be a real variety of styles at [internal] medicine, compounded by the fact that they had been working, in my opinion, too hard to see too many patients.

Not all physicians thought that they had been affected by the process of analysis; and it is possible that not all were exposed to the patient flow and straw man techniques. One Chief appeared to refer to a consulting style that had been only mildly affected by the adoption of CIS:

> I still interact with the patient the same. And I order with them and I try to include the computer, you know, while I'm standing there waiting for it to log on – and it takes much longer than I thought – you spend a lot of time waiting for the computer to log on. So I try to tell the patients: 'Well, we're just waiting for the computer to log on!' And they seem to accept it; they don't care.
>
>   I don't chart in the room. I'll write my orders in the room, but I do all my charting outside. I know that some of the doctors do chart in the room but most of us chart in our offices. So it hasn't really affected the patient care.

Process improvements were followed up with training and to some degree assessed by their impact on outcomes:

> Then the charge nurse was getting people up to speed on competencies – for example now we are saying the nurse can give more advice – is she competent to do that? And the other thing we did was to time the processes, so we did time studies – before and after the process. My role was to get efficiencies, focus on access, and we would use phone access measures and satisfaction measures and we tried to tie the processes to any measures that we could find, so that we could continually look to see if we were improving.

Alerted to problems of backsliding and coping difficulties, the team brought in an organisational psychologist:

> People were continually trying to move back to their comfort zone. So we brought

> *somebody in to talk about change management: what it feels like when you're going through a change, the peaks and valleys that you go in. And when things are happening, you could look at this chart and say, 'That's where we're at, that's why you're feeling this way – it's natural.'*

A member of the implementation team described how the analysis and improvement of existing care processes contributed to implementing CIS:

> *We spend a lot of time having pre-deployment areas document their as-is process. We've coached them a lot on how to document everything from a patient registering at the front desk, all the way through the patient's discharge. What we did with that documentation was to translate those step-by-step, as-is processes into CIS. And that was the bridge to help the users understand, 'This is what I do now: here is where I'm going with CIS'. We found that when they had no idea what their as-is was, they had no idea where they were going – it made no sense.*
>
> *We had one group that decided they didn't want to document any of their as-is, 'Just show us in CIS what this looks like.' So we did about three weeks of 'This is CIS'. Then they said, 'Time out! What do we do now?' So we had to backtrack and take them through a process to review what everybody did now, because the simple task of processing one piece of paper – people did it five different ways.*

Readiness

Specialty differences

Different specialties and sub-specialties varied in their amenability to CIS computerisation. This was due to several factors, including the nature of the discipline itself. We saw how the success of general surgery and OB/GYN with CIS was explained in terms of algorithmic disciplines – treating a clearly delimited set of problems with standardised procedures. Other factors included the personal leadership qualities of the clinic Chief and the geographical distribution of the staff within a specialty. Thus, OB/GYN was seen to have a strong, assertive leader committed to integrating OB/GYN services across several locations in the region. The relative success of paediatrics in utilising CIS, on the other hand, was attributed to its efficient organisation and release of some capacity to absorb the additional time burden.

Disciplines defined as less amenable to CIS included internal medicine, and primary care generally – an observation complicated by the fact that some primary care is given by specialists. A key factor was thought to be the greater diagnostic challenges and higher complexity faced by these disciplines. Some felt that the templates designed to help standardise charting were useless for these physicians. Internists in particular were thought to have helped design templates as a counsel of perfection instead of a practical tool. The fact that internists and family practitioners were more likely to be dealing with multiple ailments and physiological systems increased the complexity of practice and presented a greater challenge to the computerisation of clinical procedures.

One respondent saw the reaction to CIS implementation determined by the nature of the work and concomitant attitudes of staff across different locations:

Whereas [one] clinic saw CIS as a rallying point to improve low morale and a dip in patient satisfaction, [another clinic] was a high-functioning clinic ready to reject any intervention that was not a clear improvement over their current way of doing things. So it had less to gain and more to lose in terms of productivity and patient satisfaction from CIS, and was not in CIS long enough to reap the returns. Whereas [the first clinic] saw it as a culture-building opportunity, and were seeing more and more benefits, and would benefit even further from being able to access other clinics' notes online. The impact on productivity also dissuaded [another] hospital from implementing early because the region could not have two teams of underutilised internists.

The same respondent clearly saw the high-performing clinic trapped by its own performance criteria in a Sisyphean* cycle of 25 patient visits per day:

[Clinicians at one site] have really been bothered by not being able to see those 25 patients a day. They really see that as a failure either of themselves or of CIS. That's a short-sighted interpretation of what it is we are trying to do here.

The distinction alluded to is similar to that already identified between single and double loop feedback.[66] Single loop feedback refers to a system's response to information about its performance measured against established criteria, such as the number of patients seen per day; double loop feedback, by contrast, refers to a qualitative shift in how the system's performance is defined, such as when the patient-per-day criterion is rejected in favour of different ways of interacting with patients. Single loop feedback leads to quantitative, incremental change; double loop feedback leads to qualitative, radical change. To these internists, the risk outweighed the potential. They did not have a sufficient felt need to change their system of care so far as to burst the constraints that supported their conventional definition of excellence. Habituation's two main aspects are efficiency and conservation.

Another respondent explained how the basically cooperative culture at one clinic had been affected by the experience of implementing CIS:

The culture at [at that clinic] is actually quite amiable. They are mostly oriental males and, relative to a place like [another clinic], where they are much more vocal, much more outspoken, the docs at [the first] clinic are much more quiet and willing to follow orders and give leadership the benefit of the doubt. And they tried their best with CIS, but they did struggle with it, emotionally as well as technically.

We were averaging about 25 patients a day and now we're down to about 20 or 21. And they were frustrated physicians because they were willing to give the leadership the benefit of the doubt. The leadership made a big effort to explain why, but it seems they weren't willing to listen back. And that's what got docs frustrated: nobody really seemed to listen. And when they spoke out the expectation was, 'This is what we have, these are our limitations, and we are hearing you but we can't do anything about it.' And that's just unacceptable. Not for medicine – maybe for something else, but not when you're talking about medical care.

The internists were prepared to try CIS but became alienated by a perceived

---

*Sisyphus, a mythical figure condemned by the gods to the repetitive task of rolling a large boulder up a mountain, whence it would roll back down of its own weight.

inadequate organisational response to their concerns. Internists at another clinic had assessed its impact and elected not even to *try* the application unless it could be shown to be more effective and efficient than previous methods:

> *If there was one index case that really led to the demise of CIS, it was the specialist and primary care internal medicine physicians. They just drew the line and said, 'No, we're not using this. It's going to harm patient care, especially if the region wants us to keep up volume.' And access is quality of care: if you can't get into the system, that's poor quality of care. So they just drew the line and said no.*

The attitude at this medical centre also contrasted with the response at another clinic, where some physicians were eager to implement and apparently never thought to question the rollout, as another physician noted:

> *There are Early Adopters in our clinic who took leads in the CIS project. That contrasts to individuals at [another clinic], who felt empowered to look at it and ask, 'Is it something worthwhile?' I don't think we ever asked that question.*

E-literacy

Other dimensions of readiness to adopt CIS included computer literacy. This varied across sites, specialties and occupations:

> *This department is more computer literate than most departments, and because of that we volunteered to go first, knowing that it would be somewhat painful, but also understanding that we could do it better than some of the other areas. We already had a baseline skill set in the department. Like A, who is very into computers and loves diddling with gadgets. And B, who loves the stuff. And then – everyone can type.*
>
> *I found out that a lot of our Medical Assistants can't type, but I hadn't thought about that up until that point. If you can't type it's a problem. You have to dictate. Either that or you're going to get this productivity issue that comes up.*

Another Chief emphasised the role of vision and excitement in grasping the potential of electronic systems. Here we can see the implication that CIS in some way fitted into this department's perceptions of its weaknesses and its desire for better systems of care:

> *I mean we were just ready: we could just see the power behind it. Then there were users who, though frustrated by this particular application's faults, nonetheless read in it an image of a better model of care. Yet equally there were those who wanted nothing to do with CIS.*

Size

Sites differed in size and complexity. The more groups within the clinic, the greater the challenge to implement, as a clinic manager described:

> *I think the larger the group, and with multi-processes, it made it extremely difficult – when they brought them up – and I don't know if we realised, with the different roles and processes, how difficult it was going to be: 60, 70 people. There are five*

teams, each with separate leadership, versus the first clinic, which is four doctors, a tight group, great leadership.

It was a qualitative difference in the level of difficulty, because with internal medicine alone it wasn't just physicians. We had nurse practitioners, physician assistants, the RNs who do care management, and the advice and procedures; and the clinical pharmacists, the certified diabetic educators: they're all part of that healthcare team. It took many, many meetings. We worked with them a whole year.

Healthcare teams

The advent of healthcare teams was seen by some respondents to facilitate CIS implementation. Of the 26 teams in Hawaii, some specialised in internal medicine and others in family practice. Some smaller practices had a mix of, for example, one internist and three family practitioners. The general unit was: four physicians, two nurses, a nurse practitioner, four medical assistants, a receptionist, a behavioural medicine therapist, sometimes a physical therapist, a clinical pharmacist, and a diabetic educator with case management responsibility for diabetes. Exceptions to this model included a group of eight family practitioners at one clinic who had elected to be one large healthcare team. Physicians were salaried – they were not free to go and give care in other facilities. Salaries were based on the Medical Group Management Analysis Survey and the target was the mean salary for the nation.

One Chief explained how a burgeoning team ethos increased the readiness of clinicians to switch to CIS:

We have regional healthcare teams. There is a physician leader and a non-physician co-leader. The key relationship is between the member and his or her PCP [primary care provider] and the rest of the team is there to support this relationship. This was all in place; very well established; had been going on for at least five years before this [CIS] came. So they went from being traditional, individualist doctors to having to work as a team, evolving as leader of that team, and then working with data and outcome measures to improve processes, service and behaviours. So it was kind of fertile ground, 'OK, here's another tool [CIS]. How do we make this tool improve what we are doing?' So the team-based thing was really helpful.

A senior administrator also noted the contribution of teams to the implementation of CIS:

One of the really good things was that we had to start working as teams, as built teams. So we got teams to work on this. If we didn't do that we would be much more dysfunctional. Because people weren't even used to working with each other. At least now they are used to working with each other. We are very fortunate in that the team building preceded CIS.

A clinic manager reiterated that view:

I think one of the things that made this successful for Hawaii region and the peripheral clinics was that we had already had five to seven years really focusing on working together as a team.

The existence of established teams facilitated implementation because individuals were accustomed to communication and collective decision making:

> There is a big difference between established healthcare teams when implementing a big change like this and groups that are not in healthcare teams: because the communication isn't there; established meetings – just structure.

A member of the implementation team explained the specific importance of the medical assistant and physician partnership concept:

> It has made the medical assistant and physician relationship, their teamness, a lot better. Because it's usually one who is the whiz at the computer, and they are learning how to support each other. Often it's the MA that is the whiz and just knows how to get in, get out, or to find things: they've looked at it, and they're pushing their doc to 'Keep up! Keep going! Don't stop! Keep moving!' and so it's a reversal of the hierarchy.

The same respondent had also found a key difference between secondary and primary care, with primary care tending to be more advanced in team working and perhaps having a more collaborative approach overall:

> Specialty care is completely up in the air as far as a team culture. That really depends on the leadership. As a whole our region has been trying to get primary care redesign going and it really stuck and grew at [one clinic] in general. They're just more collaborative there. So that may be a part of what you are seeing.

That might have been a reflection of the region's priorities, but as the same interviewee suggested, it might also have reflected differences in medical education that the physicians had been exposed to, both in their academic and practical environments:

> In medical school they're trained that you're gonna be the one-stop; you're gonna be it, the final authority. I'm hopeful that more collaborative approaches are being investigated at medical schools.

A clinic Chief recalled how the process of team building was conducted in answer to a prevalent pathological individualism, low morale, and an absence of mutual support. The implication was that new clinic cultures and leadership styles were necessary precursors to CIS implementation:

> So before we implemented CIS the clinic supervisor and I decided we needed to bring the team together. And so we spent – this was maybe two years before CIS – a good six months developing principles of the clinic and working on teamwork and trust. Because we knew that if we couldn't work as a team there was no way CIS was gonna fly: we would just fall flat on our faces.
>
> So we spent a lot of time talking about what we do in the clinic, why we are here in the first place, why do we want to work in this clinic versus other clinics, stuff like that. It's not the doctor taking care of the patient: it's the clinic as a whole taking care of the patient.
>
> Trust and respect for each other and our patients; work and grow as a team based on honesty, integrity, compassion and dependability; strive for excellence; live by our principles in regards to ourselves, clinic and region. The whole clinic built those: the housekeeping, the front desk, the doctors and nurses, the MAs. So I think

that gave us a good basis when we had to make a lot of changes in how we do things. We had some underlying respect for each other's jobs.

'Teamness' was seen to affect how each individual site fared with implementation: a site with already functioning teams was more successful with CIS than one still operating the sole practitioner model; as one training team member had found in a comparison between a medical centre (except internists, who as we have seen refused to implement CIS) and another clinic:

They already had pretty sophisticated care models at [the medical centre]. When we started training them in 1998, they had handoffs established to all their ancillary providers; they had named teams; they really hung together and huddled. At [the] clinic there was more of a culture of practising alone together. You know, they came in, they had their MA, they worked heads down in the same clinic, but they weren't really doing a lot of collaboration. And so I think that this is making up for years of that type of practice, which is totally common in healthcare.

User responses to CIS

Training and support

The specific challenges of implementing CIS at different sites did not all arise from local structures and processes. The relative success of CIS implementation at the first clinic, and its failure at another clinic, also related to choice, with some respondents noting that the first clinic chose to go first, but that [the other] did not choose to go second. There may also have been significant differences in levels of training and support provided, as a clinic manager explains:

It was easier at [the small clinic] because they chose to go first and they accepted the mantle of what that would mean. They were well supported in terms of training and resources and time and communication; and there was a lot of reward and recognition that was built into the whole process. You did have very strong and committed physician leadership.

The department that had the most difficulty was Internal Medicine. Number one, they weren't given a choice about being the second site. I think if they felt that it was their decision and they had some choice in terms of readiness, I think they would have been more accepting. Internal medicine wasn't supported as well as the first clinic was, in terms of resources to allow the learning curve.

According to one of its members, the training team's approach to implementation was set within a wider, long-term perspective. New technologies come and go, but people still have to get on and work together:

My main concern is relationships: because this is a journey, not a one-shot deal. And so we're going to be rolling out various implementations, so we need to have relationships and trust with these people. We say, 'Area Manager (or Nursing Supervisor), here is the buffet of ways that we can do this with you. Tell us what will work best for you.'

So we've done this in a model of buy-in, communication, a lot of information, and a model of having a coordinator who says to clinic leaders, 'I am your single point of contact; I'll give you all the information about resources, whatever. This is our generic game plan and now let's fit this template over your clinic schedule; your clinic challenges, whether those are personalities or ongoing issues such as access problems at the clinic. These are my locum resources that potentially we can use and negotiate. Let's try to work this out.' So I think this model has been very successful.

One Chief complained that he was unable to train himself off-site, which frustrated doctors' customary learning methods:

A very big frustration for me too was that you could only use it at work. Which means you could only learn it at work. Imagine you're a medical student and you can't take the stethoscope off-site. You can't learn. That's not how doctors learn to use a computer. And that's another reason why it was so slow and so frustrating. They wouldn't even give us dummy patients to practise order entry with.

Most informants spoke highly of the training and support provided by the project team. However, one criticism was made of its focus on adapting clinicians to the application rather than showing them how to use CIS as a tool to change their practice.

Interestingly, implementation team members perceived a reverse phenomenon: they saw *users* being obsessed with pressing the right buttons instead of what CIS could do for them. Project team leaders emphasised the importance of using CIS, and Epic in future, as a tool to redesign practice, but reported that many users had been slow to recognise that potential. This comment by one super-user illustrates the user's perspective:

We quickly found that what we were trained to do was how to use CIS. But that isn't what we really do. So what I mean is, we were trained that 'if you hit this button, this is what happens'. But that's the least of what we're doing when we're taking care of patients. And what we weren't trained to do – and what we really hadn't prepared for as well as I hoped we would, is the thinking that, 'Your goal is to give good healthcare and you're going to use this as a tool to provide good healthcare.' The training was around 'using this tool'.

The same respondent couched the problem as *incorporating* CIS into clinical practice:

So we had a whole bunch of trainers: very good at what they do; very nice; very easy to work with; doing their very best to teach us something that they actually didn't have to spend a lot of time to teach us, because the program itself was relatively easy. But figuring out how to incorporate it into the actual care we were giving to patients – that was a more difficult task, which our trainers weren't really equipped or prepared for. That wasn't their insight, their focus. In retrospect that was a mistake. We should have recognised that; and it was part of a larger mistake when we think about CIS itself and why it was not the best solution for us.

But defining the challenge as *either* adaptation *or* incorporation arguably fails to connote the radical transformation faced by the clinicians. The challenge was not to adapt CIS to practice, any more than vice versa. Nor was it a task of *translating* the rational, digital language of information technology into the organic language of medicine, or vice versa:

They were focused on the buttons and translating their paper workflow exactly into an electronic workflow, just to get over that transition; and then finally they discovered that in a lot of the things that they were trying to translate, it was not efficient to do it the exact way they did it. They didn't even need to do that sometimes – things they had always done but there was not a lot of value to it.

Implementation team members observed different speeds and types of adaptation, some beginning with hesitation and creeping forward incrementally, others making sudden leaps forward:

There's this nervousness about learning the application and the buttons that I think users have to go through. So they want their workflow to be as normal as it can be; and then once they realise that the buttons are not that big a deal, then they start thinking, 'Oh. You know what? We don't have to do it this way; we can do it that way.' And you can sometimes leapfrog some of that, but sometimes you still have to go through some of those steps.

Aptitude

Some implementation team members expressed surprise at how much variation they had encountered in the reactions of employees to CIS:

What's fascinating to me is that you think that everybody is going to respond to an implementation in kind of the same way, and it's not – you get all these different personality quirks. And people who tend to be a little more obsessive are gonna have trouble with this; and people who are not visual-spatial people are gonna struggle with learning where those icons and buttons are. And they are going to do it all over again with Epic, even though it's a better system. [...] So that's kind of what the fun thing is: trying to find all these little individual responses to it and how do you help to support them?

Another CIS team member noted different reactions among physicians to suddenly having vast information resources at their fingertips: some searching exhaustively, others preferring not to search at all:

Now that the physicians were electronic they were doing information overload, in that they had to see every single report, every Internet website, everything they could get their hands on before they could make any kind of decision – even if it's just approving a routine medication. And then there's other people that it looks like they're saying, 'Information is going to slow me down, I'm just going to approve this stuff' – just like they probably did with paper, because to get the chart and all that took time. Neither one of those extremes is really the ideal, there's somewhere in the middle, someone that's getting enough information that there's no major risk but being able to move forward.

Other members of the implementation team reported that some physicians found CIS disruptive to old habits and routines. In those cases, one would expect a temporary reduction in efficiency, at least until the application was integrated into a revised practice style. One respondent thought that adapting to the new technology was partly a generational issue (though other members of the team did not agree). One clinic manager saw a strong need to revise their whole approach to implementing new systems on the back of Hawaii's experience with CIS. The future emphasis should not be on a mechanistic approach to learning the technology, but on changing the psychology of users, enabling them to radically revise how they practised. Nothing should be taken for granted and all the old care processes are potentially dispensable in the transition to an electronic environment. Otherwise there is a danger of automating inefficient practices instead of inventing new ones to capitalise on the opportunities electronic systems provide:

> *I definitely hope that we do Epic differently. My feeling is that if we were to roll out Epic in an identical way – having little segments of the population, and then having intense backfill, and then the idea being that you are now ready to fly.*
>
> *In many ways we didn't put a lot of pressure on changing how doctors think. We put all our attention on the technical parts of it: you need to learn how to type; you need to learn how to do this; you need to learn how to use the mouse properly. I would kind of hope that we put more emphasis upon workflow and changing the mindset. Because if we go into the same mindset, which is, 'We saw this many patients before; we're gonna do the same darned thing, but now we're gonna do it in a computerised record; but we're just going to take our paper chart and magically put it in the computer, and change nothing,' we'll fail.*

The same respondent concluded that implementing CIS was not about new technology in the narrow sense of computers and software, but about a radically new approach to health technology, in the broadest sense of all the ideas, techniques, interventions and organisation involved in the maintenance of health:

> *What we need to focus on is to change our healthcare delivery system, which is very different. And that would then make Epic a part of what we are doing, rather than in the centre and we work around it. The idea being: let's put the patient in the centre and create a better environment.*

Implementation team management

Several respondents commented on the leadership and management of the implementation team. It appeared that their resources could have been deployed more effectively. Of the three teams set up, one was overburdened while the others were under-occupied and it appeared that little was done to rectify the discrepancy until late in the rollout. A clinic manager recalled:

> *I mean we had most of the implementation sites over here, so we had probably 80% of the deployment and yet they had three deployment teams within Hawaii. They had two teams that didn't really do a lot, and our implementation team was like bombed. Only at the last deployment did they [think], 'Oh, these people over here aren't doing anything!' So then they started bringing people over from the other training teams.*

As one explained, overworked team members felt under considerable, perhaps unnecessary, strain. Let us bear in mind the Hawaiian taboo on 'talking stink' and interpret the following excerpt carefully. The halting speech at this point in the discussion bore witness to the difficulty the respondent felt (being interviewed along with a fellow team member) in being completely candid. I think that the feelings expressed may have been stronger than a cursory reading might suggest. The self-image had been bruised by participation in CIS implementation. From the tone, paralinguistic behaviour and physical appearance of many respondents, the physical and mental exhaustion evinced by this person was quite typical:

> There's been a considerable amount of stress involved with that, which in my case certainly has affected my family a little bit, as far as getting things done and keeping a balance.
>
> It's just been [pause]. It's been difficult. I think we have to look better at how we work, and at replacement hours. People go on vacation, folks get sick; folks take different jobs. How do we handle that as a team? Hawaii is so small that we don't have the latitude to say that, 'OK, if you go, I'm your partner'. There needs to be more of that built into the structure so that people don't stress out. I think that really needs to be revisited.
>
> A lot of the money goes to research and development and to the product itself, and the people part [pause]. As well as I think the Hawaii region does, we could still be better at it in terms of making sure there are replacement people – because we help each other out. But you don't even have enough time to write down everything that's in your head. Somehow we've got to leverage one another better.

There were also opportunity costs. If implementing CIS was such a resource-hungry project, what other projects had to be shelved, and was it worth the sacrifices? One implementation team member summarised the ambivalence felt towards CIS, which informed the poignant and somewhat deflated mood expressed by some of the team members interviewed:

> It's hard to know where to start. I would liken it to a roller coaster. We knew this was a really big change for physicians' practice lives. It takes a lot of organisation to get it done, so there were a lot of people and resources and things put on hold in the region to get the project done. So because of that it's particularly hard right now because of the change in the direction of the project.
>
> Even though you know it's for the best; that we're going down a better road, there's all this self-reflection about all this work we did, and all this stuff that we didn't do in the region. The stuff that we ignored for three years as we tried to do this project. So there is a bitter-sweet, 'What have we spent all of our time doing?'

The fact that certain respondents later publicly described their research interviews as therapeutic is some indication of their responses to the abortion of CIS implementation. Some appeared to mourn the project and all the time and energy devoted to trying to make it successful. This has important implications for project management. How were team members to make sense of their experience? Was it a success, a failure or something in between? We think that they, and the region as a whole, needed help to account for this uncertainty and to form a positive interpretation to support a sense of achievement and self-worth, as this excerpt demonstrates:

> A lot of what we did we will be able to use on the Epic project. But I think the sense in the region is that we have really spent a lot; and we have given up a lot in our

> *region to try to do CIS; and we won't ever get back what we put into it. I think that's the sense out there, even though we know that we are actually going to get a lot back from what we did. So I think we are trying to overcome this image of a failed project.*
>
> *I give myself about five seconds every so often to just kind of like take a deep breath; say, 'OK, it's too bad,' but there's no point in lingering on that.*

Momentous change can be emotionally, cognitively and physically challenging.[51] To what extent did the implementation of CIS impose additional demands on Kaiser Permanente employees, and what resources could they draw upon to meet them? Some demands occurred at the individual psychological level. The following quite passionate excerpt, from an interview with a regional administrator, characterises this type of challenge. The respondent is ostensibly speaking in the voice of a third party:

> *'We're going through an enormous culture change. Even though you've given me an eight-week ramp-up of training where I was seeing half of my patient load for a couple of weeks, gradually increasing my patient load. So yes, I feel like I've had skill building and so forth – but don't you understand that this has changed my whole experience of being a doctor? I can't ever be the way I used to be with patients in a room. Whether that's good or that's bad, I don't know, but it's completely upset all of my learning to be with people in the doctor–patient relationship and you don't appreciate that.*
>
> *'And how dare you say that I need to be more efficient or effective in this delivery; or that these things are somehow to make my workday easier. And, if my workday is easier, so what? I'm the delivery vehicle around here: you people just sit around and talk. I'm delivering the care.'*

Time burden

Most interviewees expressed concern about the additional time burden of using CIS. If some physicians in Hawaii already worked long hours, there could be little spare capacity to cope with the additional work required to implement CIS. Why was this obstacle unanticipated by national and regional leadership? A possible reason was that the culture of Hawaii Kaiser Permanente inhibited physicians from voicing their concerns loudly enough to be heard. On the contrary, they seem to have concealed those concerns with bravado, as an implementation team member noted:

> *The physicians in [one clinic] all give 110% and work 10–11½ hours per day, so there was no capacity for an increase in workload implementing CIS. On the other hand their attitude was very gung-ho and patriotic. If somebody comes along and says, 'We would like you to do this', they will not say 'No' – which puts themselves under a lot of pressure. That would not be seen because it wouldn't be shown. Although with CIS we did try and give some hints – when people got up and said, 'This is going to be a real challenge, but we're going to do this!'*
>
> *But you know I had these private discussions with the physicians at [another] clinic and they were very conflicted about, 'The organisation has asked me to do this. They are asking me to be successful with CIS.'*

The organisational culture may have ultimately worked against a successful implementation by inhibiting negative feedback concerning its feasibility, and by encouraging unwarranted cheerleading in its favour. Moreover, regional leaders appeared not to have interpreted correctly the doctors' euphemistic expressions of concern, such as, 'This is going to be a real challenge'. For what they actually meant was 'This looks *impossible.*'

Comments by physicians tended to confirm the impression that CIS implementation and use imposed a significant extra time burden, and that the additional cover provided during the settling-in period only deferred the problem, as one physician noted:

> *It was not an easy rollout for any of us and we're still having a lot of difficulty. We all dread April 1. We have backfill that has been provided for us. On first of April [2003] we lose that backfill, so the big question is, 'What are we going to do about it? How will we handle it?' At each clinic people are developing contingency plans for 'What if we* can't*?'*
>
> *I would see 24–26 patients in an eight-hour day. In our regular clinic functioning we are expected to handle, let's say, overloads – patients who can't quite fit in our clinic schedule, and currently they are being handled with assistance by an extra locum because of the CIS program. So come April 1 we lose that extra help and we're expected to handle the pre-CIS load.*

Reduction in access to care was another problem raised by the extra time burden of using CIS. The Chief of another clinic raised this problem explicitly:

> *You know, we couldn't see as many patients as we did before. So for six months we had an additional FTE [full-time equivalent] here, and we just lost that person because they pulled the funding. So now we're not sure what we're going to do, because we used to see a full schedule plus overloads. We can't see the overloads anymore. Even if we want to we can't physically do it because it's just taking more time.*
>
> *Right now we're at a crossroads. Now what are we going to do, because we don't have this extra body to help us to see all the overloads? And how are we going to accommodate our patients? And we're not quite sure what we're going to do.*

The overloading problem was also raised by a specialty Chief:

> *Operational efficiency is a major issue. The entire department is understaffed. So we see large numbers of patients per physician. So efficiency becomes a major issue. What do you need to get the day done; what do you need to get out of here on time – or not dramatically overtime – became a real issue. So what you don't need is a new IT system that doesn't overtake tasks that you were doing before, and gives you extra work, and adds a learning curve on top of that.*

Couching the problem in terms of operational efficiency gave an insight into how that Chief viewed the culture of the department, but also how added pressure can tend to confirm and retrench a culture of blind efficiency, possibly leading to a breakdown; or even becoming a catalyst for change.

A department that values operational efficiency might tend to assess its own performance mechanistically, responding to new external pressures by focusing even more intensely on achieving established, preset targets. Which is perhaps why, albeit tongue in cheek, the same respondent suggested an absurd alternative to recording every clinical action electronically:

> For the cost of CIS you could hire someone to follow the docs around to record everything they say. Some feel that introducing IT into healthcare turns the doctor into a clerk. Does it make sense to pay 10 times as much for the doctor to transcribe his own notes?

The logical conclusion of an efficiency culture pushed beyond the limits of its endurance is breakdown: a catastrophic loss of integrity such that it can no longer function according to its established rules. This is apparently what happened to some CIS implementation sites. The outcome was a realisation that the old ways of delivering care were not viable with CIS, and some were fatally flawed anyway, as this Chief noted:

> We certainly said, 'Well, I'm gonna work harder; we're gonna stay later; we're gonna get over this hump and such,' and we discovered that we really couldn't. We had started out in the high ninetieth percentile in terms of our utilisation, so when we tried to add the constraints of the system, basically it broke.

On a related point, another specialty Chief had found that CIS had improved the standard of notes as they had become accessible to a wide and possibly critical audience:

> On a bad day we might see 30 patients. There's no way that you can do that on a computerised system, unless you're going to do as lousy a note as possible. And most of us have too much pride to want to. It's surprising how often you look at it; even people who don't type well are going back and correcting their typos. And all of this takes more time. You don't want to put out a bad product...

Though no one identified *spare* capacity in any clinic or department, it was evident that some were more overstretched than others, as one Chief suggested:

> I think there definitely are differences among clinics. For example, [one clinic] indicated that, 'No problem, we're back to business as usual.' But when you really talk to the people there, it's not really business as usual: they are working a heck of a lot harder than they were; plus, their utilisation [percentage of available appointments taken up] was not high. It wasn't low, but it wasn't in the mid-nineties like ours was. We had a lot of overloads [patients without appointments] in our system that balanced out people who didn't come – it's kind of like the airlines [standby]. And there were some days when everybody showed up [plus the overloads] and it was really not that pleasant. I think [they] had a little bit more leeway in their schedule, so they could absorb that. We couldn't.
>
> But even [at that clinic], if you talk to the Chief, he indicates that he couldn't keep up this pace. I mean it would definitely drive him to an early grave if he saw this as never-ending.

One Chief provided some specific examples of how CIS had impacted on clinic life:

> Recently, I've managed to get out on time but for the first three or four months I could not get out on time, and for 11 or 12 years prior I never left late; never,

never left late. And for months after we went up I was here 30, 45 minutes later and that was really hard for me, because I have young kids and I have to go get them, you know I had to pick 'em up by a certain time. And everybody else has stayed late; everybody has stayed an average of 30 or 40 minutes later than they used to, or else come in early.

And now everybody works through lunch. They never used to. You know everyone used to sit at lunch and we could have a talk. Everybody works through lunch now. It's taken a significant toll on time.

Now we are in our offices, charting. So we never talk to each other any more. We used to be able to stand at the counter and write and maybe, 'Hey, how're you doing? How's the day been? How're the kids?' But we never see each other anymore because we're either in a room seeing a patient or in our office charting. So I kind of don't like that. That's just an aside that I noticed. I think that's important for collegial and camaraderie stuff.

But we do OK in this clinic because we built it up beforehand, but if we didn't have that I think everybody would just be off on their own.

The additional workload imposed by implementing CIS had wider effects on capacity too. For example, it may have delayed the ability of clinicians to innovate in ways that CIS could have supported and in other ways, as a member of the implementation team noted:

I think that there was so much work to be done to incorporate the tool into their workflow that, frankly, as process improvement oriented as our organisation tries to be, still our primary mission is to see people who need our help. And they've had some access issues over there; getting people in and frustrations over some people not being able to see their primary care physician. So I think they may not have been able to move as full speed ahead as they would like to with process redesign, because of time.

The impact of previous IT innovation

We asked about previous electronic medical records implemented in Hawaii Kaiser Permanente. According to one senior administrator, CIS had been the fourth and most ambitious electronic medical information system implemented in the region:

We had a very small start with IBM in the early 90s as a project that about four or five physicians took on. Then, more recently we implemented a product called the WAVE that is used by 12 internists and the Medical Centre, and [by] a group in the neurosciences department: the neurosurgeons, the neurologists and the physiatrists use this WAVE product. And we really call this the first major system that's being used, and it's being used today. There's a second system that is not a user system in terms of daily practice, but is actually a clinical reminder system called the Population Care Registry.

However, it was unclear exactly how successive systems overtook previous systems in practice. We suspect that there was no common pattern across sites. Wide variations were reported in how systems had been used in different clinics and departments, and a similar level of discretion allowed when new systems were implemented. This had perhaps resulted in a unique configuration of utilisation at each site, and a most uneven pattern of usage across the region. A member of the implementation team attempted to explain:

> *We started with the WAVE documentation system. That got pulled and then we went to a very safe product, the population care registry, which was initially intended to complement an electronic medical record that was going to have nine components from nine different vendors. Then we ramped up to do CIS. Rough dates are: 1998 for WAVE, 1999–2000 for Y2K, 2000 PCR, and then for the last two years we've been doing CIS. I think we will start our deployment of Epic January 2004. That's very fluid.*

No study participants reported 'fatigue' from successive implementations. Indeed, most viewed EMR adoption as imperative to deliver more efficient and higher quality care, as this Chief noted:

> *Going from paper to a computerised medical record is probably the big step. So we took a big step to go to CIS, and it'll just take a small step to get to Epic. So we don't think it'll take us very long to change to a new medical record system. And we knew that whatever we changed to could only be better. It couldn't be any worse.*

However, some respondents referred to employees who were not among the believers. None of the latter was interviewed, which could suggest a sampling bias, but probably only by self-selection. One member of the implementation team perceived a range of attitudes among employees on the desirability of electronic systems:

> *People had various degrees of understanding and belief that you really had to do this; that you had to go to electronic systems. They saw it in the context of that belief.*

A clinic manager gave the specific example of internists already working with WAVE and who were sceptical about the potential gains offered by CIS:

> *[One clinic] already had WAVE. They had already gone through this process once before, so they were cautious. They were going to watch the process.*

Arguably, the most significant impact of experience with previous electronic systems was imported from *outside* the organisation in the shape of the new Kaiser Permanente CEO, as a key member of the implementation team described:

> *Our Medical Director, to his credit, kept feeding back that this is not a good product. But what really changed it is that they got a new CEO at the top of the organisation, and he had gone through the same process in his previous organisation. And he had come to the same conclusion. They had embarked on a process, as I understand it, that they were going to build their own – something similar to CIS, and they realised that it didn't work and they actually stopped that and went to Epic.*
> *If they had selected a different Chief Executive, I don't think we'd be where we are. I think it was one guy and he happened to have that particular experience. And he said: 'Hey, I've been through this: this ain't the right decision.' If they had picked anybody else we'd still be with CIS.*

This suggests that despite the problems encountered trying to implement CIS in Kaiser Permanente, the project had acquired sufficient momentum as to be unstoppable *without* a change in leadership at the very top of the national organisation. This also raises questions about the ability of an organisation to change course after it has been set, despite the internal communication of important information about serious problems and concerns with the system. Why was that? What are the characteristics of some organisations that prevent them from interpreting information constructively? Or is this an attribute of all organisations? What are the internal political commitments that maintain a course of action that no longer appears justified or rational? It is unlikely that this effect could be explained in terms of organisational structures or even processes. It is more likely that an inability to change course has to do with the sort of cultural dimensions that have been raised in this report: culture, leadership, approach to implementation and capacity for change.

Resistance

The implementation team saw overt and covert resistance to CIS. This was difficult to manage in a non-hierarchical medical culture. Resistors might simply put themselves at the back of the queue; they were almost at liberty to deselect themselves from the program. Even harder to address were those who agreed to implement but did not follow through. We have noted the imperative taboo in Hawaii Kaiser Permanente – the preference for polite suggestion over curt commands. The normal and symmetrical response is to accede, to be agreeable. But there is an important distinction between agreement and agreeableness, which if missed might result in concordance more formal than actual, leading to considerable frustration for the project team. Criticism of others ('talking stink') is proscribed and, since negative assessments of CIS might imply criticism of sponsors, constructive feedback was suppressed. As a result certain parts of the organisation, while publicly assenting to CIS implementation, did little about it privately, or may even have tried to actively subvert it.

We have noted many reasons for individuals and groups to be disaffected with CIS, including its technical shortcomings and high rectification costs; and the disagreement and dysfunctional communication between different levels of the organisation. What causes of resistance to implementation were articulated by respondents? One source of resistance (and we recognise that resistance may have been unconsciously as well as consciously motivated and expressed) was the awareness by e-literate employees that better products than CIS were on the market. It was deeply frustrating to have to participate in the implementation of an inferior system, as this regional administrator noted:

> *Now the problem with CIS was: it was such a huge change and the functionality wasn't there to make it easier for the physicians, and so we encountered a lot of resistance. And in the meantime the national organisation made some directional things, like, 'OK we are committed to CIS, we are going to make this work.' And at the same time people have heard that there are other applications that are better, that could make the physician's life easier because the functionality is there. And then there were these things about, 'Well why couldn't we get CIS to function in those ways?' And CIS wasn't mature enough to do that.*

One physician identified the main source of resistance as individual:

> *I think they ignored the male physician surgical ego and didn't think we would question them.*

But one Chief implied that resistance ought to have been anticipated as a structural feature of relations between national Program Office and Hawaii:

> *Program Office is basically the organisation that deals with dollars, and harsh reality-based decisions like space and staffing. So when a mandate comes from Program Office the expectation should be that it will be resisted: not that people will just smile and do what they are told – especially not physicians.*

The resistance was ultimately vindicated by events. But whether CIS could eventually have worked in Hawaii, we will never know for sure.

Conflict

Conflict was reported within and between different levels of the organisation. Clinic Chiefs and project team members were torn between their knowledge of CIS's faults and their responsibility to promote it in the region. Hawaii Kaiser Permanente's clinical interests were seen to conflict with the financial and administrative interests of the national organisation. Conflict was perceived between Kaiser Permanente's need for tailor-made software and IBM's need to produce a marketable product. Finally, a significant proportion of behaviour described by respondents could be classed as conflict avoidance. Against a conflict-averse Hawaii Kaiser Permanente culture, some admired the willingness of leaders to tackle the national organisation over the deficiencies of CIS.

Personal conflict

Personal conflict was implied in most interviews and expressed openly in some. One Chief found himself in the dilemma of leading his clinic through CIS implementation, when he realised its adoption had been a big mistake. The parallel drawn in this excerpt between leading a clinic into CIS and troops into Vietnam is potent, not least as the interviews were held during the opening weeks of the 2003 American-British invasion of Iraq, in a climate of tension, uncertainty and fear.

> *There was a faction of people who felt strongly that CIS was not the best option for us; that it was a mistake to go with CIS. And in retrospect I have to say that they were right. They had looked at other programs; they thought that the func-tionality of CIS was not state of the art. And so as a clinic Chief I'm heading towards trying to get my staff ready for this and I'm being addressed by people whom I respect saying, 'This is a mistake: you should do what you need to do to stop this before it goes on,' and I felt very conflicted then.*
> *I felt like I was an officer asked to take my troops to Vietnam and people are telling me I should go to Congress about why we are going to Vietnam. You know, that may be true but my focus needed to be on making sure that my troops survived*

and did well. That conversation about 'Should we get into Vietnam or not?', that was supposed to have been addressed long ago.

By this time the strategic decision had been made to go with CIS. I trusted that this decision was thought about really hard, and they were making the decision on valid principles, and they were trying to do what was best for the organisation, which included me and my staff and especially my patients. My thinking about this was, 'Well, so maybe it isn't the most functional system but we're hooked up with IBM for Christ's sake, and if IBM can't help us, who else can fix this?'

Another Chief reported a similar internal conflict between the role of dutiful leader and personal reservations about CIS:

I think that another Chief way back in the beginning said: 'It's like working with a bad Medical Assistant. It's better than not having one, but sometimes it drives you crazy.' And I really thought it was going to be a lot easier to chart on the computer than it was. I kinda like technology stuff, I'm on the computer at home, and I can type pretty fast and everything, and it was really cumbersome and I was really irritated with it. So, on a personal level I had to kind of, um, bite my tongue to try to lead the rest of the clinic through it.

Regional–national conflict

Respondents often referred to the importance of voicing one's concerns and being listened to. Not to listen was evidently offensive. This was congruent with a culture that, in contrasting itself with the US mainland, took pride in *not* listening to those who shouted loudest. Softer, more nuanced voices need sensitive hearing. Hawaii Kaiser Permanente expected to be listened to carefully by Kaiser Permanente national, and was disappointed. Seemingly, national and regional expectations of CIS were different and conflicting, as one Chief analysed:

And when we look at cultural issues, the impression that I got regarding the decision to go with CIS: I think that the highest priority was not usability; was not, 'What's going to make the clinician's day easier, or more efficient?' It seems that the highest priority was, 'How can we document as completely as possible and then extract information easily, so that we can get paid, and so that maybe we can do research?' but had very little to do with taking care of the patient who comes to your office.

Another Chief reflected on his own assumptions about the national organisation in terms of a critical distance between Hawaii Kaiser Permanente and Program Office:

What I saw as a weak point of CIS was, for lack of a better term, Program Office; and I refer to them almost as an entity out there, like the IRS [Internal Revenue Service], like the Government. I don't think Program Office realises how the average frontline physician is somewhat alienated by them. If you add on top of that a heavy-handed mandate from Program Office – that this is coming down, and you will implement it; then ignoring local leadership and their opinions on the culture of the local environment in rolling that out, it's a formula for failure. They ignored the communication chain and just went straight for the jugular. There was no foreplay, so to speak.

In this narrative a blundering Program Office is contrasted with Hawaiians' need for sensitivity and consideration. Perhaps their differing expectations of CIS, and of one another, were underpinned by different unspoken assumptions regarding the proper way to disseminate innovations. Program Office was seen to view CIS as instrumental in meeting the organisation's financial objectives; whereas Hawaii Permanente physicians expected to be seduced into compliance. One can reduce the analogy to a fundamental logic that is normally neglected by technical approaches to organisational change: the logic of rites and ceremonials. We know that rites and ceremonials play a central role in organisational life.[68] We have demonstrated in this account how ritual elements of Hawaii Kaiser Permanente culture mediated implementation of CIS. Examples include the ritual obtaining of consensus in decision making, leadership rituals in the posture of support for CIS, even when conviction was lacking, ritual deference to the individual autonomy of physicians. And when one considers the consequences of departing from these rituals, one immediately sees how intimately they are involved with the functional side of organisation, for instance that a heavy-handed approach to coercing physicians to implement would have provoked a highly dysfunctional response.

But it would be unsafe to conclude that Hawaii Kaiser Permanente culture is more ritualistic than Kaiser Permanente mainland culture. Such an ethnocentric assumption implies a primitivism without any empirical basis. It could be argued more convincingly that an instrumental approach to technology innovation is just as ritualised as a consensual approach but has merely forgotten the ritual basis of its procedures, whereas in Hawaii ritual still tends to be acknowledged.

The same respondent then switched to a more instrumental lexicon, but grounded his argument in a conflation of good medicine and the financial health of the organisation. In the last sentence we note again what at first reading might seem an innocuous criticism: that CIS had made nice people 'talk stink'. But if talking stink is taboo in Hawaii, something that makes good people act *so* badly must itself be a very bad thing. This can be read as a euphemistic condemnation of Program Office, with which CIS was identified. In this way the Chief effectively names Program Office as a perverse influence on amiable doctors to such a degree that they transgressed normal standards of behaviour: they talked stink:

> *Program Office had prioritised financial outcomes, a return on their investment. They had to, that's their business. And I guess we saw things differently: if you want to see a return on investment, there is no greater return on investment or financial security than just practising good medicine. That will return back manifold. And you're not helping us to practise better medicine, you're forcing us to take shortcuts; you're forcing us to document things that don't need to be documented; you basically turn doctors into order entry clerks. And, yes, that reduces human error, but in the big picture of things, how many times is that a human error thing? And they had to compromise their values and ethics to help the system work. And that's where I saw very amiable, nice, quiet people starting to talk stink behind the scenes, and they're just very frustrated by it.*

Although that passage is emotive and its assertions dubious (sadly, it would be naive to think that practicing good medicine is necessarily the best return on investment), it doesn't really matter because the truism it contains remains potent: Program Office made some nice doctors talk stink; pushed them over the edge.

One implementation team member also blamed the highest echelons of the Kaiser Permanente Program:

I think the problems that we had with the national organisation – and it may not be their fault because they were constrained – their priorities were to get something rolled out under a certain budget, in a relatively short timeframe. They had difficulty dealing with being told: 'Hey look, you gotta fix this because it really makes it hard for users.' And because of those constraints they really weren't set up to deal with that. And to an extent they didn't understand it. And to some extent their hands – the people making the decisions – were tied by people above them that were driving money, you know, very high in the organisation, that were focused on budget.

'And to an extent they didn't understand' draws attention to a theme developed earlier: that national and regional organisations were operating within different paradigms, or cosmologies. As Mary Douglas observed, each primitive culture is a universe to itself.[18] She might have added that every culture is primitive in the sense of being concentric or inward looking. Perhaps, assisted by information technology, globalisation will finally destroy all 'primitive cultures'. Hopefully not.

Conflict between Kaiser Permanente and IBM

Another paradigm difference seemed to dog relations between Kaiser as customer and IBM as vendor. This was especially significant as Kaiser Permanente physicians played an important role in specifying certain CIS functions, including templates designed to facilitate recording of clinical data generated during the patient visit. So the 'very unexpected changes' which this respondent refers to were partly changes to Hawaii Permanente physicians' own specifications, an indication that involving users in software development may be more problematic than might be imagined:

So there were those types of failures, the classic systems failures where 'This is what we want' tossed over the wall to the developers after we thought we had a clear understanding: wait, wait, wait. Developers toss it back over the wall and say, 'This is what you asked for.' You know and it didn't work. It didn't work. And then these folks become very suspicious of these folks, and its like, 'Well what is your job, you know, as it relates to this product?'

Physician involvement was also made more difficult by the lack of a working example of CIS in which to ground the development work. That, as one Chief explained, presented a huge obstacle to specifying detailed procedures and templates, which were to some extent outdated by the time the software finally arrived. The solution? IBM delivered templates designed for another region. It would be easy to underestimate the importance of this lack. Not only could it have prevented physicians from realising their templates visually and dynamically, on-screen; it would also have rendered their work abstract in the sense of not having any empirical cues, frames, checks, or reinforcements. They would have been working, as the saying goes, 'in the dark'. More precisely, the lack of a working model would mean that their templates were theoretical and with little if any consistency with the CIS software. Small wonder, then, that the templates IBM delivered were rather different from those the physicians thought they had designed.

We were interested to learn where respondents thought the blame for this problem lay, with IBM or Kaiser Permanente. In fact, respondents were reluctant to attribute blame to IBM, and more inclined to blame Kaiser Permanente. For example one implementation team member blamed Kaiser Permanente for approaching CIS as an internal development project:

> I don't think the contract between the vendor and the purchaser was the problem. Basically, CIS was an internal development project for Kaiser. The fact that IBM was the vendor really didn't change the fact that it was still an internal development project, and that basically Kaiser was establishing their requirements, and IBM was responding to those requirements. IBM is not in the healthcare industry. The bottom line is, IBM is still a manufacturing company. They do some software development and custom application design and development for customers. But that puts all the pressure, the onus and responsibility on the customer to decide what they want in a product. It was no different in the CIS project.

Not every respondent held such crystalline views on who was to blame for the failings of CIS, as the following excerpts from two different interviews illustrate:

> I've heard that the relationship with IBM was not very good. We wanted to make a whole lot of changes and they would point out why it would take time and cost money, and the smallest change would be a fight and it would cost tens of thousands of dollars. It seemed to be a very confrontational relationship, as opposed to a cooperative relationship.

And:

> We really felt like we knew healthcare best. But we don't know IT best. In hindsight we really do healthcare better than IT.

Conflict between medical and nursing staff

Finally, one member of the implementation team referred to conflict between medical and nursing professions regarding scope of practice issues. This implies that nurses' awareness of working out of scope was an incipient source of conflict between themselves and the physicians. As we saw in the section on scope of practice violations, the 'reality of the business' was that some nurses were acutely aware of practising on the borderline between nursing and medicine, but may have felt unable to refuse physicians' requests to take on contentious tasks. In this case, the nursing-lead would welcome a resolution of conflict between practice and licence, whereas the physician-lead might defend an apparently satisfactory *modus operandi*.

Conclusion

This chapter paints a nuanced, multilayered experience of CIS implementation, to which the application of a curt lexicon of success and failure seems quite inadequate. If we, along with Kaiser Permanente, are to learn from this experience, we should resist the urge to close the case prematurely; proceeding always to the next innovation, never looking back in case of what we might see. Is this a vain hope? Generally, researchers look backwards and managers look forwards. Learning from previous implementations requires a bridge to be built between these two opposite trajectories. If managers want to learn from past work they must be prepared to cast an objective glance backwards; if researchers want to influence practice they must cast a pragmatic eye to the future. This is a familiar lament, and a vain one as long as researchers and managers are motivated by different reward systems.

Chapter 4

Barriers and facilitators to implementation

Chapters 2 and 3 examined participant experiences of implementing CIS in Hawaii Kaiser Permanente, and how they explained and accounted for that experience. We also began to articulate a critique of the familiar and, it would appear, facile binary opposition of success and failure. It now appears irrational to summarise such a complex reorganisation of working relations and routines as, simply, one or other; success or failure. There is a world of difference between summary judgements, which seem intent on closure rather than disclosure, and the vivid experiences of implementing CIS.

We mark the passage of events symbolically, and perhaps this ritual function is what terms like 'success or failure' mainly serve. And if there are rites of implementation, there are also rites of evaluation. This is not to empty evaluation of its substance, or relegate it to a formality. Moreover, as noted in the previous chapter, we delude ourselves and debase our culture if we think that our innovations are empty of ritual. Being strange to our eyes, the rites and ceremonies of Hawaiian culture, as they inform innovation, stand out sharply; whereas our own are largely invisible to us. We should awaken to the fact that our customary emphasis on *performance*, which refers variously to financial, human and technical efficiency, is in itself ritualistic. Which is to say that it is socially valued and marked. Indeed, so hyper-ritualised has performance become, that we almost completely overlook its obviously dramaturgical reference. Efficiency is no more or less than a socially enacted value. One lesson to learn from Hawaii, as the cultural context of this research, therefore, is to remember ritual and ceremony in its important function as a kind of cultural grammar, analogous to linguistic grammar, and necessary to the articulation of change. Each act has a double quality of substantive content and ritual significance, being instrumental and expressive in one and the same motion.

We therefore begin this chapter with a summary of our findings in terms of *multiple* successes and failures. It will be seen that no grand conclusion can be drawn from this summary. Each success or failure is a nuance, a reflection glimpsed within a net of jewels,[43] in which each nuance reflects others and cannot be viewed in isolation. The different ways that respondents accounted for successes and failures are then also summarised, along with the barriers and facilitators to implementation explicit or implicit in those accounts.

Summary of findings

We begin by deconstructing CIS implementation from a mythical unitary entity into an actual plurality of events and processes as evidenced by the interviews. Rather than persist in attempting to decide whether 'it' has been 'a success' or 'a failure', we enumerate many failures and many successes in an attempt to add a realistic texture to an evaluation of CIS implementation in Hawaii. We see now that there is no unitary 'it' at all. Implementation is always already multiple and complex. At this intermediate point we retain the basic binary opposition of success and failure in order to demonstrate not only that any unifying judgement as one or other would be spurious, but to also show a paradoxical element in their relation to one another. In particular, that a 'failed' innovation can 'successfully' trigger other innovations.

Failures

- The adoption and implementation of CIS was controversial, contested and resisted, from the outset.
- The software was delivered over a year later than planned.
- The product had certain technical deficiencies and was slower than paper to work with.
- The substantial contribution by Hawaiian physicians to the software specifications was frustrating and ultimately wasted.
- One influential group of physicians refused to implement the product until such time as they could be convinced of its superiority to existing systems.
- Getting changes to CIS was unacceptably slow and expensive, deepening the disappointment and frustration of users.
- Problems were systematically collated and reported to Kaiser Permanente Program Office, which then set its interest in billing against the physicians' interest in usability.
- The process of implementing CIS penetrated almost every activity in the region, hugely increasing the workload of the implementation team.
- Many existing customs and practices were incompatible with CIS, including failures to update names on licences to practise.
- Medical assistants and registered nurses were found operating beyond the scope of their licences.
- Physicians were obliged to document patient care more fully, eroding their use of verbal orders.
- Certain functions of CIS were especially problematic. The electronic In-Basket appeared to have been designed in partial ignorance of how physicians actually managed lab test results. The templates were relevant only to less complex sub-specialties that would least benefit from their use.

Successes

- On the other hand, CIS spurred innovation in some unexpected ways.
- As an additional burden to a system already struggling to cope with demands for access, CIS forced Hawaii Kaiser Permanente to begin to find alternative ways to deliver care.

- *Inter alia* CIS convinced many of the advantages of electronic medical records, particularly those stemming from a readily accessible, up-to-date patient record.
- The dysfunctional In-Basket prompted revisions to lab results management, relieving some physicians of unnecessary work.
- Exacerbation of access problems combined with the availability of an electronic record prompted various experiments to improve access to care, including MD telephone triage, team visits and even more radical ideas concerning the sacred cow of the visit.
- Whilst some of these initiatives had already been aired in Institute of Medicine and Institute of Health Improvement reports, they had not really fallen on fertile ground until CIS both increased the burden and provided inspiration to challenge accepted practice.
- CIS improved physician accountability by imposing an external demand to maintain more detailed records usable by other clinicians.
- More widely, the inter-clinical nature of CIS created a new regional infrastructure for decision making.
- Clinic and sub-speciality Chiefs began talking to one another and became capable of participating in collective decisions across practices.
- Communication with outside agencies also improved, and more discrete and portable documents, such as referrals, could be handed to patients to take to the visit, or sent to nursing homes.
- The foregoing successes relate to quality improvement for patients but also to organisational security and risk management.
- Practices related to State licensing, Federal agencies, and clinical auditing were exposed and corrected in the course of trying to implement CIS, leaving the organisation legally, ethically and financially more secure.
- CIS was well received by Kaiser Permanente members, who saw it as a sign of modernisation, improved communication and continuity of care.
- The patient flow and patient straw man process studies specifically aimed to improve quality and efficiency of care and were an integral element of CIS implementation.
- Improvements in chronic disease management were modest and only partially attributable to the CIS patient record function, but still contributed to the start of a more systematic approach.
- Other lessons learned from CIS included recognition of a need to focus on the human as well as the technical characteristics of system use.
- The importance of preparatory work in advance of implementation was appreciated.
- And the uneven texture of the organisation was recognised in terms of differences in readiness and ability to implement across and within individual clinics and departments.

The adoption decision

The quality of the decision to adopt CIS was seen as one reason behind its failure. Specifically, Kaiser Permanente national HQ was blamed for making incorrect technical and financial assessments. With Kaiser Permanente bearing all development costs, CIS was, with the benefit of hindsight, seen to have been financially doomed from the start. There was an assumption that if CIS worked in Colorado State, it would also work in Hawaii. Several reasons were offered to invalidate that assumption. The two regions had different organisational cultures, Colorado was more authoritarian and Hawaii more consensual; Colorado had big call centres, which Hawaii had rejected; Colorado had 20-minute and Hawaii 15-minute appointments; Colorado did not have similar access problems to Hawaii.

It was thought that inadequate advice had been given to those responsible for the adoption decision by management consultants. Partly as a result of this, HQ had failed to analyse properly the logical, technical or financial implications of the contract with IBM. IBM also made mistakes, by failing to foresee some of the problems associated with co-opting doctors into the design process; or research adequately how the physicians practised. Take the In-Basket function: seemingly, IBM did not understand how doctors actually managed their lab results. It did not know, or take into account, that some Registered Nurses were practising on the fringe of medicine. So these informal practices – how the organisation really worked – were not accounted for.

Nor did Kaiser Permanente apparently realise the implications of its dependency on IBM as sole CIS customer. IBM could charge what it liked for improvements because it had a cornered market. Kaiser Permanente locked itself into that hostage position, which only an executive decision at the very top could reverse. In fact it required a change of CEO to halt the implementation.

Was the consultation with Hawaii region adequate? Apparently not: some of its most senior technically competent medical staff did not like CIS and did not think it could work for them. This information was systematically discounted or ignored.

Respondents were slow to blame IBM for the failings of CIS. They saw the fault in the contract, and in Kaiser Permanente's myopic faith in a company renowned for its hardware but lacking a similar reputation for software innovation. And it was seen as Kaiser Permanente's fault to commit itself to bearing all the software development costs.

Technical problems

At this point one might be tempted to try to identify rules of engagement to guide future, similar programs. But we find that such rules tend to slip through one's hands, at least with regard to Hawaii Kaiser Permanente's implementation of CIS. Let us first think about the technical problems encountered. Some of these may have been effects of direct and indirect organisational causes. Decision making in large organisations can be complex, even irreversible, in the sense that it is impossible to reconstruct it accurately. We did not have access to the original decision makers, some of whom had left the organisation. Respondents did not view the problems encountered with CIS as purely technical: they were intimately involved with the culture, leadership, differences between specialties and between primary and secondary care, training and support, aptitudes, etc.

Actually, the technical problems with CIS were inextricably interwoven with the whole adoption process: priorities, research, financial forecasts and so on. Plus, clinicians were involved in some of the design work. Parts of the application were imported from Colorado State, where they had been designed for a different organisational setting. It seems clear that the technical specification and functioning of CIS was at no point in its development ever a purely technical issue. That the technology was a factor in the career of CIS in Hawaii is banal and undeniable, but only conceivable in the wider clinico-socio-cultural context of Hawaii Kaiser Permanente. There is no simple independent technical variable here.

Approaches to implementation

How CIS implementation was approached influenced its career in Hawaii. An awareness of dissemination research helped in the choice of implementation sites.

The extent to which the advantages of a heterogeneous approach to implementation were foreseen, or learned along the way, by reflecting on successes and failures, we do not know. But it was clear that administrators and trainers had a sound knowledge of the region's localities and personalities. This supported an informed choice and order of implementation sites – a choice that tried to include the preferences expressed by participants. An alternative would have been to plan the implementation according to strictly rational-technical criteria, allowing no choice. That might have worked better or worse, we cannot tell. However, those charged with the implementation clearly perceived an unevenness of readiness and willingness across the region, which they were wise to exploit rather than to ignore. We think their responsive approach was less risky and took advantage of a degree of local knowledge not available to external consultants or contractors.

Sub-specialty differences were also seen to influence different levels of success at implementation sites. These differences can be analysed into the technical and the institutional. For example, one high-performing clinic struggled with CIS because it had high utilisation and no slack. But it also struggled through having a 'we-are-a-high-performing-clinic-with-no-slack' mentality. Schein advises the organisation therapist to hunt out discrepancies between espoused values and behaviour in order to reveal unspoken assumptions.[85] It was arguably the high-performing clinic's own perception of a threat to its system's integrity that caused it to revolt. Internists believed in their duty to maximise access and saw that CIS would erode their performance. The basic logic informing decisions at the clinic appeared to have been that care depends on access to the clinic; CIS threatens to reduce access: therefore CIS is an enemy of care. As they were soon to learn, however, it all depends on how access is defined: access does not have to mean a *visit*. By beginning to define access less narrowly, the clinic began to discover new ways to resolve their conflict between the EMR and quality of care.

Smaller clinics were more agile, partly *because* they were smaller and had a bit more slack and partly because they had Chiefs more switched on to e-health. But if their size mattered, it was not the only factor. Equally important were vision and a commitment to aims that escaped the confines of syllogistic thinking – to thinking, as the trite but apt phrase has it, outside the box. Which is another term for double loop feedback.

Training and support

Trainers found that some users were ready and eager to transform their clinical practice with CIS, whilst others plodded painfully through its basic functions and struggled to assimilate it. This uneven pattern of learning between users, and between sites, challenged trainers at first, but they reportedly learned to adopt flexible training and support strategies. They also located some limits to that flexibility. For example, one clinic signally failed to implement CIS *without* analysing its workflows and care processes. One wonders if all the tacit knowledge accumulated within the team will be properly valued and exploited. After the traumatic implementation of CIS some members might have been tempted to return to practice or move on – which could be a great loss to the Epic program.

Analysing the workflow and patient journey was essential to implementing CIS and had far-reaching benefits in terms of a sharing of practices. Needless to say, this was also an invaluable aid to implementing future systems, both for the substantive gains in efficiency and to demonstrate the value of the technique.

Specialty differences

The characteristics of different clinical specialties offered varied challenges to implementation. Relatively linear, algorithmic procedures, like those of general surgery, were more amenable to CIS, whereas internal medicine and primary care presented complex barriers to computerisation. This suggested a need for a simple and flexible system. CIS appeared to have been too prescriptive. It did not allow users enough choice at the basic level of how they could use it. Most physicians did not use templates because they were cumbersome to use, especially in multiples. Perhaps CIS offered more advantages in terms of financial coding, but Hawaii Permanente physicians were less interested in that aspect than in the quality of care. The real incentive for physicians to use CIS would have been to save time *and* improve quality of care. Not that the physicians can have been entirely indifferent to billing. It did pay their salaries and bonuses after all.

In CIS different sites saw different challenges and opportunities. To some it was viewed as a threat to a record of achievement they were not prepared to sacrifice. To others it became an instrument of clinical integration. To still others CIS imposed a welcome discipline which providers had been unable to impose on themselves. CIS was not the same system to everyone, therefore, and the variety of interests it could potentially serve was perhaps a facilitator or a barrier, depending on whether an opportunity was perceived and grasped. The decline in morale at one clinic could have inhibited uptake of CIS, but was construed instead as a condition amenable to improvement. At another clinic, CIS could have been seen as a potential tool to help internists escape the treadmill of patient overload, but their collective attitude was such that it was perceived a threat. The point is that, at any site, reasons could have been found to implement CIS or *not* to implement CIS – and they could have been the same reasons viewed from different perspectives. Attitudes are basically very simple, being either positive or negative; their valence is not beyond conscious decision.

A great magnifier

Hawaii Kaiser Permanente came to recognise the folly of organisational intervention without close analysis: prior to, during and after implementation. *Inter alia*, the organisation achieved a much better understanding of the care actually delivered by different clinics and practitioners. And a purge of unnecessary differentiation in practice was found necessary and valuable. CIS involved a microscopic examination of care processes. Automation demanded standardisation, which in turn required frank communication between practitioners. This resulted in some previous idiosyncrasies being modified or discarded. But the wider lesson to be learned is the magnifying effect of CIS implementation – that any EMR would be like a lens held over both good and bad clinical practices; and that, once addressed, the bad would generate a considerable amount of additional work to correct.

It was found that certain irregularities in names, licences and local working practices delayed the implementation. But these were only raised *by* the implementation. It would be perverse, therefore, to characterise such irregularities as simply barriers, and more accurate to argue that CIS usefully revealed these issues and led to their resolution. CIS brought a new mode of supervision to medical practice, a new visibility, which allowed people to see what individual physicians were doing and asking their staff to do. Some welcomed this, aware that their practice administration could be tightened up. Let us say then that some of the informal routines that develop in any healthcare organisation are potential barriers to EMR implementation, but may be revealed as barriers only with the change in circumstances and processes that innovation demands. In other words, the habits formed under one regime may become vices under another. Changing systems involve revisions of the familiar as well as the shock of the new.

CIS team management

The aforementioned additional work, which included a lot of organisational firefighting and policy making, threatened the integrity of CIS training and support teams. Resources were not optimally deployed, as one team was overstretched and two others relatively idle for several crucial months. Doubtless the unwillingness to complain did not help the unlucky overburdened, but the main lesson is surely about more active supervision and management of the implementation/support team.

Whether the CIS team's management could be said to have aided or impeded implementation is a good and valid question that cannot be answered by this study. This issue brings an overall theme of the study into sharper focus. In discussing successes, failures, barriers and facilitators to implementation, we are actually addressing two different and related concepts. On one hand is the program itself and, on the other, the 'health' of the organisation. To pronounce an implementation a resounding success when the sheer effort and conflict involved leaves the organisation exhausted and demoralised is paradoxical. A judgement of success or failure must include both concepts. What we really want is full implementation of a program *and* a healthy organisation. What we found in Hawaii Kaiser Permanente was an organisation under siege to CIS. Threatened thus, employees became worried about the health of their working community as well as the health of its clients. In the example of the implementation team this came out clearly. Some of the team members appeared exhausted, and admitted that trying to implement CIS had been a 'wild ride'. For some of them the balance between achievement and wellbeing had clearly not been managed as carefully or successfully as it might have been.

Nothing and everything to do with CIS

Outdated names on licences, scope of practice issues; unnecessary and inefficient heterogeneity of practice styles and procedures: these caused an escalation of work for the implementation team. The thing to note here is that what made the organisation work – its informal aspect – disrupted implementation of CIS, partly because roles inevitably drift and formalised interventions have to cope with such discrepancies. Slack should be built, therefore, into budgets and timelines to manage the informal organisation. Formal and informal structures and processes enjoy a complex relationship of mutual adaptation or symbiosis. Changes to formal structures and processes disrupt that symbiotic relationship. An organisation is a relationship between its formal and informal aspects. Perhaps that complex relationship is the real unit of analysis and intervention.

Unsurprisingly, in view of their very clear focus on the relational character of social organisation and health, many Hawaiians saw and expressed a relational perspective when they coined the phrase 'It has nothing to do with CIS and it has everything to do with CIS'. Nothing to do with CIS because it was not specified in the blueprint; everything to do with CIS because the blueprint is just a two-dimensional plan which reveals nothing of its actualisation or conduct. As soon as the plan began to be implemented, the living organisation was affected and reacted. Informal practices were therefore a barrier to CIS implementation in one sense. But in another sense they were the very preconditions of its implementation.[67] No innovation works by virtue of formal plans and procedures only: there is always a heavy draw on the will, energy and commitment of those whom it affects. None of this is in the blueprint, it isn't even recognised. It is a well-hidden cost. Without that extra hidden effort, no innovation would work.

The time burden

Every respondent except one testified to the additional time burden imposed by CIS. The burden reduced over time but was never likely to disappear. This was a very serious concern, which, surprisingly, one senior administrator dismissed as trivial. Clearly communication and understanding broke down on the issue, which is likely to recur with subsequent interventions, including EpicCare. The time burden was an effect of several poorly designed functions and probably did more to delegitimate CIS than any other factor. CIS extended the duration of the visit and delayed access to care by some members. That was unacceptable to physicians in Hawaii. It wasn't just the turning away of patients, or working even more hours, but a threat to their self-image and reputation. Hawaii took pride in being the most highly rated Kaiser Permanente region on certain metrics, including patient satisfaction, and was most unhappy about that reputation being damaged. To that extent at least, CIS threatened not only the region's performance, but also its identity.

Change imposed on top of overwork and coping difficulties is likely to increase stress. Demands to change may be ignored or paid lip service if no possibility can be seen to incorporate them into an already intolerable workload. Or such change may lead to some form of breakdown, or revolt. Because CIS added time to the work; because this was not adequately addressed; because this was predictable, one has to ask 'Why?' Surely the five-minute difference between appointments in Colorado and Hawaii should have been accounted for. Hawaii's shorter visits could have been a major barrier to success with CIS. Leaders should have heeded euphemistic warnings, like: 'this is going to be a real challenge'. One of the barriers to CIS implementation was simply time. Physicians hadn't enough time for it. It took up too much of their time – it was self-defeating. Computerisation should mean cutting the time to perform routine tasks; and time is a key element of competition. An electronic application that does not cut time, or actually lengthens tasks, is a contradiction. It is perhaps fruitless to speculate as to whether later applications will prove less of a time burden, as the context was altered by the CIS implementation. The challenge now, a more optimistic one, is not to perform the same visit in less time, but to redefine the visit, which includes redefining the time and place *of* the visit.

Healthcare teams

Hawaii Kaiser Permanente was fortunate to have promoted team working prior to and as part of CIS implementation. Without that experience the whole business of people sharing how they did their work would have been even more problematic, and the benefits in efficiency less than achieved. Of course, solidarity can also yield resistance, as one clinic demonstrated. But it is reasonable to suppose that less progress would have been achieved if each site had to be approached as a collection of individuals. It appeared that, through CIS implementation, clinics became even more integrated and coherent centres of care; and that certain sub-specialties achieved greater integration across clinics as well.

Organisational culture

Respondents placed a high value on their organisation's culture. They attributed some of the successes and failures of CIS implementation to the anti-authoritarian medical culture. Key concepts of *aloha* (love) and *ohana* (family) were pervasive and appreciated by both recent settlers from the mainland, and by more established Hawaiians. The guiding principle of the *healthy relationship*, between Kaiser Permanente and its staff, and between the staff and the members, provided policies and practices with an ethical mooring. Kaiser Permanente has never been an organisation adrift on the ocean of fee-for-service medicine. The marketing slogan 'Caring for Hawaii's people like family' was not empty rhetoric, but a sincere value statement conveying that, although *in* the market, Kaiser

Permanente was not entirely *of* the market. The package offered was not just healthcare *per se*, but membership of a family in which health was maintained and cared for in a distinctively Hawaiian way.

Hawaii Kaiser Permanente staff therefore sought ways of achieving efficiency that would preserve their provider–member relationship. On one hand, it could be said that a failure to implement CIS fully in the region was partly due to an absence of command and control leadership in the medical culture. On the other hand it could be said that the organisational culture survived the rigours of implementation because it held relationships above technology. However it was, the coup de grace for CIS was delivered from the new Kaiser Permanente CEO, but it was a blow long wished for by some influential Kaiser Permanente staff.

Each clinic or sub-specialty mediated the implementation in the sense that the locale, the people and their subculture adapted and modified the software to their needs. Initial sites were chosen according to their status as innovative, early adopters and followers; simple or complex; large or small; indispensable or dispensable. And the factors defining each clinic as an institution, including all the non-operational factors, were as important as the operational characteristics of the medical work involved. The utilisation of CIS at each site depended on a number of factors, each having both structural and cultural facets. OB/GYN, for example, saw itself as performing clearly definable procedures and having a strong directing mind to ensure implementation. But it also had an OB/GYN culture, which may not be as aggressively individual as some surgical sub-specialties. The primary care context in particular proved an unreceptive environment for CIS to thrive in.

Dissemination research guided implementation, by choosing likely sites and by relying on demonstration and reference groups. Should that strategic approach to implementation be viewed as internal or external to the organisation's culture? Probably the former. Arguably the way an organisation reflects on its own profile and behaviour is central to its 'personality'. This was certainly the case in Hawaii Kaiser Permanente, as all respondents were explicitly concerned with issues relating to the kind of organisation they worked for, its style and ways of relating to members. It did not seem to occur to them that they were involved in an unquestioning adventure to maximise revenue, or access, or any other single outcome. What mattered was achieving the optimal balance between these factors, the healthy relationship.

We also saw that Hawaii Kaiser Permanente's culture influenced the assessment of success or failure by its reluctance to criticise. Whether the implementation would have been more successful with the benefit of more candid feedback from users and others is impossible to say, as every other aspect of the context would have also been as different as between Hawaii and Colorado, for instance. A more decisive assessment of CIS might have been achieved in a shorter timeframe in another region than Hawaii. But whether the context of a different region would have been sufficiently comparable to prove the application for Hawaii – as Colorado was thought to have done with an earlier version – is debatable. The lack of clear answers to these questions underlines the idea of innovation as relational. It is neither the application nor the context, but an unpredictable co-mingling of the two.

To posit organisational culture as a facilitator or barrier to CIS implementation may be erroneous. A culture is liable to be disrupted by a new technology. To treat the organisational context as an independent variable in this relationship seems almost bizarre – shouldn't CIS be the independent variable and culture the dependent one? When prescribing a medicine, its effect on a patient's condition is what we are interested in, not the patient's effect on the medicine. Actually, this appeared to be how our respondents viewed the implementation. Of course they were concerned about success or failure, but their ultimate concern was with the organisation that they worked for. Perhaps, then, in light of the findings, we should revise our original question to address the impact of CIS on Kaiser Permanente and not vice versa.

Then can we speculate about specific aspects of the organisation's culture and CIS? Not usefully, we suspect. Where practices, beliefs and assumptions surfaced and resisted change, it was generally because they were challenged and this was likely to happen in any culture. The bottom line is that staff and members of Hawaii Kaiser Permanente did not want their culture *or* the technology; they wanted both together, seamlessly. As for the implementation team, they were in it for the long term. Technologies, even classes of technologies, come and go, flow through; but ultimately one still needs to get along with one's colleagues and members.

Nor is it helpful to think about changing sub-specialty cultures or clinic cultures at specific sites. As one administrator put it, if you look after your employees, the rest comes naturally. CIS, like call centres, or potential employees, was put to the ultimate test: what was its impact on the provider–patient relationship? What improved the relationship? The electronic health record, for example, was valued. What did not improve the relationship was discarded. In other words, the culture triumphed, which with a healthy culture is how it should be: the global process should not be radically altered by a specific, transitory intervention. There is too much at stake to gamble an organisation's culture on one wave.

All of this is vaguely disturbing as it disrupts our assumptions about causality in innovation. We tend to forget that the innovation itself is not the subject. This displacement of the organisation by the innovation is due to the interests invested in the new and expensive, rather than the old and established. What surely matters is the performance of the whole system. All technologies are dispensable from that perspective.

Leadership

Respondents valued the non-directive style of medical leadership in Kaiser Permanente. Here, too, it is impossible to say whether a more directive style would have eased implementation. Some CIS team members thought that it would at least have helped them to interact with implementation sites more effectively. But a more forceful leadership might equally have pushed resistance further underground, widening a deficit between rhetoric and action.

Another leadership style might have ensured fuller implementation, but would the sites actually have used the software any more than they did? Fear of censure would not have improved the application *per se*. A more directive style could have eroded the same trust within the region that probably made it an ideal context for a tried and tested application like Epic. At least Hawaii only rejected

CIS: it did not reject the implementation team or the regional leadership, either of which might have occurred if the faulty product had been forced in where it was unwelcome.

The situation was in any case more complex, with wrangling between Hawaii and Program Office, and the millstone of improvement costs slowing down development. The laissez-faire leadership style may have led to a more thorough testing of CIS than an authoritarian approach, as the application had to sink or swim on its own merit at each site. It was after all primarily an innovation in software, not leadership, though it ultimately tested both.

Another relationship where more forcible leadership might have been beneficial was that between regional and national leaders. Some respondents, whilst supporting the efforts made on their behalf in that arena, would have liked their case even more forcefully argued, though they also thought that lessons had been learned by regional and national offices from the experience. To most respondents what mattered was to be *listened* to.

Respondents attributed the failure of CIS in part to a perceived ambiguity among leaders, caught in a dilemma of needing publicly to support implementation whilst privately doubting its viability. For them, the decision to abort was a vindication. But here we see the paper-thin line that innovation treads – it could all have been so different. Direction from the top could have been reinforced, the implementation effort reinvigorated, difficulties overcome, and the whole story of CIS rewritten in more positive terms. The ultimate fate of the system might have hung on the insight and experience of one or two individuals at the top.

Of course, there was diversity among leaders and attitudes to change. But Kaiser Permanente leaders were deemed to have learned from the episode, especially clinic Chiefs unused to thinking inter-clinically; unused to leading at all in some cases. Hence, CIS indirectly led to a transformation in the region from clinical leadership as implicit, titular, even reluctant ('When they asked for volunteers I was just slower than everyone else to take one step back'), to a more active role in decisions affecting the whole organisation. It became possible for the organisation to take collective clinical executive decisions, possibly for the first time.

Was the leadership style in Hawaii Kaiser Permanente a barrier or facilitator to CIS implementation? There is no simple answer to this question either. Consensual leadership was seen to slow the pace of implementation and provide ample opportunities for doubters to resist it. But we cannot separate the style of leadership from the culture, or indeed from the structure, of the organisation, not at least without simultaneously raising some of the unspoken assumptions that form the main structural supports of the institution: a process more frightening than any new technology to some participants. For example, it is assumed that as professionals, physicians must be allowed a high degree of discretion in their work. A command and control style of management is incompatible with that. It is assumed that Hawaiians are offended by being ordered about and that they will respond to such rude treatment in ways that could be far more damaging than a stand-up argument, soon forgotten. Beneath the face-saving assent may be hidden a deeper erosion of trust and cooperation.

So we see leadership style not as a separate entity, but more as a mode of conduct that emerges through complex interactions between the actions, beliefs and assumptions of those who would lead and those who might be led. The actions or inactions that we label as 'leading' are not always a result of conscious individual decision making. It may be more a sensitivity to a specific situation arising in a specific cultural context. In fact it could be hypothesised that leading is a largely unconscious response to events; a response to which accounts of leaders and led stand in a most uncertain relation. Take the analogy given by one Chief of leading troops into Vietnam: the leader is too involved in planning and logistical problems to think about how to lead. Afterwards, he might report that he did such and such for certain reasons, but in a narrative reconstructed from the memory of raw material – the experience – itself interpreted moment by moment, possibly without any adequate criteria to decide what to do. The experience and the account are not and could not be the same.

Like the officer in Vietnam, leaders in Hawaii were uncertain: is CIS viable? Can it work – in time, or can it never work? Should we sound the advance or retreat? Should we show or conceal our doubts and concerns? Leadership is a role after all. The internal conflict felt by Hawaii Kaiser Permanente leaders, about taking their staff into a campaign with an uncertain outcome, showed as ambiguity and indecision. And perhaps some of that was deliberate. Perhaps leaders were sometimes conveying a clear sign: we lead you into this because we have to, not because we believe in it. And the consumers of this message responded appropriately: they were cautious, exercised discretion about what to use and what not to use, ever watchful for a signal to retreat.

We conclude that leadership is not an independent variable for CIS implementation. It is a type of intelligence (with all the nuances of that term) to guide implementation, respond to exigencies, with many visible and invisible restrictions on its scope of action. Had CIS been a really good system, constructive criticism of a leadership that failed to implement might be appropriate. But as CIS was not a good system by nearly all accounts, it is hardly appropriate to blame a leadership style for its failure. We should rather look at what was achieved substantively and in terms of learning for the implementation of Epic, and ask what it was about the leadership that facilitated those achievements. And we would arrive at the same themes: consensus, sensitivity, advocacy behind the scenes, a certain studied/unstudied ambiguity. As one Chief said:

> I have to respect the leadership. I think they see that the folk in the trenches are working really hard, and we need to change the system for us to survive. In that sense, I really don't think CIS was a failure because it made us rethink things.

Resistance

Rogers and Shoemaker attribute resistance to innovation simply.[64] Those with power will resist any innovation that does not serve their interests. Those without power cannot resist innovation. Hawaii Kaiser Permanente physicians are powerful but salaried. Their interests do not relate directly to their incomes but to their patients and their time. CIS did not increase their incomes but it did tend to decrease their disposable time and/or the quality of their care. Where time and care were most threatened, most resistance was found and vice versa. Resistance is not always conscious. We cannot know just how much of the difficulty encountered with CIS was due to resistance. But we found a continuum between total resistance and total acceptance. Between those two extremes it is reasonable to surmise that a whole scale of resistance grew up around the implementation of CIS, feeding upon myth and rumour as well as upon fact. Was it all because they chose the wrong product? In hindsight it does appear so. And yet, as one implementation team member asserted, if the CEO had not changed, Hawaii would still be struggling with CIS and perhaps better solutions to its problems would by now have been found.

In summary, resistance was a major impediment to implementation and expressed in a variety of ways, from outright refusal to passive non-compliance. Yet Hawaii Kaiser Permanente is hardly a militant organisation. Once again we need to consider not only the effects but also their causes. The main causes of resistance appear to have been as follows:

- the fact that CIS was seen to be inferior to other products
- a sense of not being listened to by those higher up
- organisational factors, including access issues
- the time and cost of software changes
- a sense that job performance was being threatened
- technophobia.

These were arguably the real impediments, not the diverse manifestations of resistance that they provoked. All were preventable or treatable.

Impact of previous information and communication technology implementations

In general we did not find any implementation fatigue, and respondents remained enthusiastic about the next system, EpicCare. Perhaps some objectors were kept away from interviews, though we have no evidence for that. And perhaps they would have preferred to remain silent than 'talk stink' to a stranger 'sent' from the mainland. Unlike previous systems like WAVE, a perverse advantage to CIS was that few if any were likely to cling to it once Epic became available. Some clinicians, including those in OB/GYN, had capitalised on selected functions. But even among its strongest advocates CIS had mainly whetted appetites for a really *good* electronic system.

Another benefit of CIS was that much groundwork had been done in terms of dealing with issues like scope of practice; developing methodologies for workflow improvement, decision making and communicating with Program Office – a lot of these things have been addressed, paving the way for EpicCare.

Conflict

Whether conflict accounted for successes or failures depends on the organisational level referred to. We think that internal conflict was a failure factor: it caused additional stress and mistrust and appeared to leave behind a sense of loss and exhaustion. Yet little appeared to have been learned about the personal conflicts experienced. With regional–national conflict it was different: there was a sense that Hawaii region had asserted itself and had gained the confidence to do so again in the future. This is good if assertive regions help the national organisation to avoid similar mistakes. If every region pays for investments it is reasonable to expect each to contribute to specifying what is purchased. Perhaps Kaiser Permanente HQ will adopt a less paternal attitude to the Hawaii region, and perhaps Hawaii will find a stronger voice, after CIS. In the process of negotiating priorities for improvements, Kaiser Permanente national and Hawaii may have come to a better mutual understanding. Doubtless different interests remain, due to their structural positions, but there was at least a sense in the interviews of a renewed respect for national leadership, and that Hawaii was now being listened to.

Lessons from the conflict between Kaiser Permanente and IBM have also been learned. New national executives had already found that to build such a system was a mistake. Hawaii's experience with CIS reaffirmed that lesson. Hawaiians had also discovered new limits to their abilities: they were not software programmers but clinicians, and it had been a mistake to blur the boundaries between those roles. They had learned that it is hard to hold the vendor to account if you compromise your own position as customer by getting too deeply involved in designing the system. The contract itself may have been faulty if it did not maintain a clear enough separation between client and vendor. Kaiser Permanente is surely a more 'expert' customer after CIS.

Conflict was a motif running through all of the interviews: internal conflict due to incommensurable demands on time and loyalty; between internists and regional leaders over a dubious application; between clinic cultures; between old and new ways of working; between different conceptions of care; between regional leaders and national Program Office; between Kaiser Permanente and IBM; between recording and coding of care; between research and practice; between the rollout and problems of training and support resource deployment. Not open warfare but a series of skirmishes distributed throughout the region and beyond on multiple levels. A guerrilla war that perhaps became so familiar, so much a part of the fabric of organisational life as to become almost normal. There is surely something heroic about an organisation that, after all the setbacks and pitfalls met with on the CIS journey, still endured as a coherent and integrated culture. The application failed but the organisation survived and actually became stronger and fitter. It is by now a familiar meta-theme: conflict neither helped nor hindered CIS as such. It was a refining fire, through which the application was tested and would continue to have been tested if it had not been withdrawn by the new CEO.

Success, failure or learning experience?

We know from dissemination research and from numerous high-profile system failures in recent years, that for Kaiser Permanente to commission a bespoke electronic medical record system was a high-risk enterprise. It could not know in advance what exactly would be produced. Delays in delivery, technical problems, internal resistance and a developing organisational context should all have been predictable by anyone familiar with diffusion research. But, as Latour writes of Diesel's engine and personal computers, innovative products do not hit the market fully formed.[44] The 'finished' product is a result of negotiation with sponsors and markets. Yes, Kaiser spent around $800 million on CIS but, arguably, it had learned what kind of system it really wanted and how to recognise that system when it saw it. Kaiser became a well-informed customer in the market place at a time when much better products were available and it thereby jumped ahead. Whether it has an advantage over its competitors, who sat on their hands waiting, we cannot say. Some might point out their original preference for a product from Epic, the same vendor that Kaiser eventually ended up with after CIS. But we should not ignore two factors relating to that hindsight: the differences between products were perhaps less marked two years earlier; and the basic decision between buying and developing was then not so clear. Whether the $800 million was wasted or invested is a moot point. It not only brought Kaiser Permanente from a state of semi-e-literacy to a position of considerable expertise, but also took it through the experiment on behalf of the whole Kaiser Permanente system. One might shudder to think of the eventual cost of an attempt to implement CIS across the whole system, and speculate how long it would have been burdened with such a 'turkey'. CIS turned out to be a pilot for Epic, perhaps. One's thoughts then turn to NPfIT in the UK, and its £20 billion projected budget.

Wider implications

The CIS experience was not only an education in IT in healthcare. Its effects on processes of care were potentially far-reaching and profound. Physicians saw a future in systems that would enable them to redesign the visit, simultaneously generate data on individual patients and populations, build researchable databases, and secure proper remuneration for the services they delivered.

CIS was not easily assimilated into existing practice styles. This was turned to advantage, however. It forced clinicians to revise their practices; to standardise what should be standardised and reap efficiencies; to consider different ways of doing what they did. In short, as one respondent put it, CIS opened the door to the consulting room, which had previously been the domain of the individual physician. This innovation in itself has a potential to revolutionise medicine in America, and in the UK and elsewhere. Apart from patient confidentiality, which is not at stake here, what positive reasons could be advanced for the individual physician not to disclose to peers or employees what occurs in the visiting room? A less clunky, more physician-friendly system than CIS might not have prompted such revisions or led to innovations in team visits; might not have pushed Hawaiian doctors to question the sanctity of the visit itself. The slowness of CIS may, paradoxically, have helped accelerate such reforms.

Chapter 5

Electronic medical record systems: lessons for implementation

State of EMR implementation

Information technology innovation remains a major challenge to healthcare organisations. Despite a considerable amount of advocacy for its uptake, few studies have yet found convincing evidence of positive effects on health or financial outcomes. Even so, some large health systems, such as Kaiser Permanente and the Veterans Administration, have invested heavily in EMRs in the USA. The largest of such programs is currently in process of implementation in the UK National Health Service.[1,28] There are undoubtedly important inter-organisational lessons to be learned from these initiatives. However, it is difficult to generalise and apply such lessons across organisations. What works, or does not work, for one organisation might not have a similar fate in other settings. When attempting to transfer learning between organisations we should take care to compare their contexts and ecologies. An intervention's success or failure – as far as those terms have any validity – might owe as much to the organisational context as to an intervention *per se*.

The move to EMRs is based on promises to date unrealised. The EMR will make records more legible, complete, and comprehensive. It will permit evaluation of quality of care, clinician performance, and patient needs easily and inexpensively, and thus facilitate the improvement of care at lower costs. This potential can, however, only follow a lengthy and challenging process of re-inventing the way in which medical care is delivered.

In this chapter we offer tentative guidance on how to approach EMR implementation effectively. We do this with trepidation, fearing that it may be taken out of context. The danger of reducing complex qualitative data, such as this study has generated, into take-home messages is fourfold. First, all such statements tend to regress to a mean of generality, such that advice from different studies looks similar even where it differs in detail, and thereby loses much of its force. Second, the take-home message tends to suggest a level of facility that may delude the reader to underestimate the difficulty of the challenges faced, and their solutions. Third, take-home messages suggest a McDonaldisation of research. This not only abuses the level of accomplishment involved in generating good research data, it also puts pressure on researchers and funding bodies to engage in research of a quick-and-dirty variety that lacks the rigour to generate valid knowledge. Fourth, recipes for success tend to assume a high level of equivalence between different organisations. In fact, even within sectors there can be great heterogeneity between organisations, each one demanding a specific approach to innovation.

The real lessons of this study are to be gained through reading and reflecting on the detail of the earlier chapters. We highlight a few points of guidance here, but they are not proposed as a checklist for success. No one can anticipate the ideas a person may have whilst reading a text. If we could, literature would be entirely composed of instruction manuals. Fortunately that will never happen. The following pointers intend to direct the reader thoughtfully backwards, not heedlessly forwards.

Key processes

The term 'process' is used here to devalue the idea of discrete factors with determinable effects on EMR implementation, in favour of the notion of complex interactions between decisions, expectations, responses, software developments, learning, coordination, etc. Each process is interlinked with other processes. The following observations about these key processes are offered to stimulate the thinking of policy makers and managers as they approach the challenge of implementing an EMR in any organisation.

Choosing the right EMR for adoption

Hopefully, the immense difficulty in making a best choice decision in this context should by now be evident. EMRs are complex systems that we propose to insert into even more complex systems called organisations. These difficulties lie in understanding which key challenges are to be addressed by the EMR system, which potential systems are available, selecting the best system for a particular organisation, planning and implementing that solution, and evaluating the innovation (along with the processes of selection, implementation and evaluation). The CIS program has suggested a strong need to involve users in design discussions at an early stage, and during the preparation of any detailed specification. This should go some way to avoiding a specification that departs from users' own identified needs. An alternative and probably more effective arrangement would be to expose end-users to a number of working EMR systems in an attempt to locate a design that best matches their needs. We noted that this was done when a Hawaiian team visited North West and Colorado regions to see Epic and CIS, respectively. Despite preferring Epic, CIS was the system chosen for development, apparently for technical reasons. Perhaps physicians' preferences were not given sufficient weight to persuade Kaiser Permanente to pursue the technical limitations of Epic as tenaciously as they might have done. Though not offering any guarantee, therefore, the arguments for including clinicians from the earliest stages of considering an EMR are nevertheless compelling.

Dealing with initial software design problems

However rigorous and inclusive the adoption decision may be, there are bound to be some initial problems with EMR software applications. Some will be seen immediately, others may become evident over weeks or months. Whilst one would expect fewer problems with an established EMR system, differences between organisations and sites will lead to problems of adapting software to clients and vice versa. Whilst these problems are to be expected, their precise nature and form may not be anticipated. Though hard to quantify in advance, some accommodation in terms of capacity and skills needs to be made to deal with issues as they arise.

Managing impact on clinician productivity

Innovation carries with it an important element of learning, not least when habitual work routines are disrupted. But managing the impact on clinical productivity does not refer only to supplementing the workforce until efficiency is regained. The impact on clinical productivity begins with the anticipation of disruption and the emotional and psychological coping issues that will arise. This is followed by a considerable amount of learning involved in substituting new working patterns for old. Finally, the impact on established patterns of coordination between carers, and between carers and their patients, should be adequately accounted for. These multiple effects add up to a considerable burden, which should at least be anticipated. In the case of CIS, there were widely differing perceptions of how difficult it really was to return to previous productivity levels. Given the will to do so, the ability of users to return to pre-implementation productivity seems a reasonable indicator of a system's effectiveness. To implement an EMR that reduces productivity for more than a few months must prompt serious concerns, and trigger an enquiry as to why this was happening.

Managing changing clinical roles and responsibilities

In addition to changes in clinical productivity, the implementation of CIS was associated with altered clinical roles and responsibilities. This is a potential effect of other EMR systems, in other organisations. As for many other consequences, some of these role changes are unpredictable. In other words, *there is a strong empirical component to implementation.* Innovation without a strategy for the adequate provision of spare capacity, contingencies and reserves is plain folly. Innovation is premised on broad systemic change. The notion that new systems can be plugged into older systems, without the occurrence of disruptive and potentially revolutionary effects is surely naïve. What some physicians in this study saw very clearly was a deeper need to change the ways in which they organised and delivered care. This was for some the main attraction of an EMR in the first place. Of course, there were other reasons that were 'necessary but not sufficient', including catching up with technology, access to up-to-date records, etc. But the most compelling reason to adopt an EMR was, we think, a vision of what might be possible with the new technology, in terms of developments in care delivery that would not have been possible without an EMR. This was also the cause of the most intense frustrations felt by physicians: that CIS was not efficient enough to make the changes that EMR technology dangled tantalisingly before them.

Managing frustrations, resistance and conflict

How should those frustrations be managed? And what of other negative effects, including resistance and conflict? Such reactions are inevitably concomitant with planned organisational change. In the case of Hawaii Permanente physicians, considerable tolerance was shown. However, less sympathetic methods of obtaining the compliance of nurses were referred to. Steps were taken in Hawaii to help employees to orientate their reactions within a normal sequence of reactions to change. But more could have been done. Frustrations could have been allowed a better airing. Resistors could have been listened to more carefully. Conflict could have been investigated more fully. This isn't a counsel of perfection, but a call to take full individual and corporate responsibility for actions. At the very least, a debriefing process should have been undertaken in order to vent and listen to some of the pent up emotions that CIS left behind, especially within the implementation team.

Anticipating culturally informed responses

The original hypothesis behind the proposal to undertake this study was that an organisation's culture mediates between policy change and actual change. In other words, organisational culture is accountable for the *implementation gap* – a shortfall between planned and actual change. This is a question of considerable theoretical and empirical interest and has helped to inform what was investigated and written up here. That this research was conducted in Hawaii might lead one to expect sharper cultural contrasts than would be found in a less culturally diverse setting. But we should be cautious about drawing firm ethnographic conclusions. One of the pitfalls of researching in an exotic culture is to delude oneself into thinking one has understood 'it'. This is, of course, the ethnocentric trap that social anthropology struggles with. One advantage to be gained, however, lies in reflecting on one's own culture. In the chapters above we have reported some effects of Hawaiian culture on CIS implementation. But one of the most important lessons can come through a comparison of the researchers' values and the researched culture. In Hawaii Kaiser Permanente, the quintessential Hawaiian values of *aloha* (love), *ohana* (family) and *hanai* (extended family) were used explicitly to help account for how CIS was implemented. This is such a different narrative from what we might expect to find in mainland America or the United Kingdom as to give pause for reflection on our own dominant values, assumed, espoused and actual. One cannot help but feel some admiration for the Hawaiian ethos, subordinating as it does technical considerations to a culture of familial love; and some shame at our comparative lack of humanity. How cold and mean we appear by comparison.

Promoting responsive leadership

Leadership played a complex role. National and Hawaiian leaders disputed CIS development priorities. The latter struggled personally to demonstrate commitment to CIS. Implementation team leaders were stuck with implementing a 'turkey'. Many in Hawaii Kaiser Permanente must have felt uncertain, 'Do we really have to do this?' Each site responded differently and each was perceived to have been strongly influenced by its leader. With such heterogeneous responses, it seems impossible to generalise about the role of leadership, other than to affirm its importance as a key mediator. The Chief Physician in Hawaii was a focus of intense scrutiny and a key influence on implementation. He apparently decided to let CIS succeed or fail on its own merits. That strategy carried risks: a real test required regional commitment, strong sponsorship. But in the background he lobbied national HQ to address the problems with CIS. How did Hawaiian physicians interpret this apparent contradiction? Some perceived it at the time and doubted the wisdom of compliance (might CIS be withdrawn?); some might have interpreted their Chief's behaviour as inconsistent – was he being straight with them? Was anyone? One interpretation is that regional sponsorship of CIS was carefully managed: in both its strong and weak aspects, calculated to give the system a fair trial, and no more. The Chief Physician was an avowed convert to EMR technology but he was not prepared to let Hawaii fall victim to a bad system. If CIS was not viable it would not be propped up indefinitely in Hawaii.

Leadership continues to vex and elude scholarly attempts at classification. It remains as slippery today as it has been for scholars throughout the past 50 years.[70] Leadership has been determined as innate, learned, situated, distributed and consumed.[68] Doubtless all these theories contain kernels of truth. We do not intend to rehearse them here. On the strength of this study we cannot comment on whether the types of leadership exhibited were innate or learned, but they were certainly situated, distributed and consumed. Situated, as the implementation called forth a variety of behaviour intended or perceived as leadership; distributed, as each Chief and clinic manager had a different take on the innovation; and consumed, as some respondents placed a high priority on the styles of leadership observed and preferred. We suggest, therefore, that any organisation considering implementing an EMR ask what kinds of leadership will be most conducive to different stages of the adoption and implementation processes. At the adoption stage, strong technical and financial leadership should be brought together with leaders from across the clinical disciplines. During implementation, a flexible approach to leadership is needed, capable of responding in a sensitive manner to the opportunities and pitfalls encountered along the way. Of course these comments should be unnecessary, as good project management should always pay equal attention to the human as well as financial and technical sides of enterprise. This is especially applicable to the challenge of implementing new IT in healthcare, where physicians still reign. As one respondent put it, there was no foreplay. Physicians apparently expect to be wooed, not coerced, into submission. The whole history of Kaiser Permanente supports this view.

Implementation models

Most IT innovation models attempt to account for implementation failure. This is a stark reversal of the usual publication bias. It is also a warning of how common and perplexing these failures are. Sauer's triangle of dependencies model focuses on the role of the project organisation (the implementation team) to develop and maintain an information system.[1] Aarts and Berg add a fourth dimension to the model. It optimistically depicts the information system (IS), the project team, the hospital organisation and the medical staff, all working in a synergistic relation to one another. But perhaps the most interesting aspect of Aarts and Berg's model is their incorporation of a general user definition of successful IS implementation as, 'the capability to create a support base for the change of (medical) work practices induced by the system'. This is reflexive definition. Here, the broader aim of IT innovation, as seen by users, is recognised. Success, however nuanced, is associated with changes in work practices. Within that broad aim, the more specific function of implementation is to support users to make changes in their working practices *that the process of innovation induces*, whether those changes (which are further innovations) were intended or unintended. Hence, as with CIS, innovation can trigger a chain reaction of innovation which the implementation process must then support. It was precisely the attempt to support such unexpected changes that overextended the capabilities of one out of the three support teams set up in Hawaii. This is also why dynamic leadership and management of the implementation team, to deal with unexpected workloads that spring up as the rollout occurs, are so important.

Complex adaptive model

What is this process of innovation? CIS implementation demonstrated the behaviour of a complex adaptive system. We would argue that no independent variables were discernible. Though we have of necessity analysed the results of our interviews, the time has now come to synthesise those variables or factors back into a more holistic model. Decisions, adaptations, clinical specialties, personalities, culture, leadership, etc. all bleed into one another; none exist in abstract. Each, as it were, exists in one another. Each reflects the others as in the fabled net of jewels.[43] We can state, therefore, that these are really not factors but key processes, not very clearly defined, which are interdependent, contextually dependent and ambivalent. The flux of organisational life and transformation is not like categories on a page, but like the ocean, constantly in motion, with changing winds, currents and swells.

Catching a wave

Which nautical reference leads us back to the preface to this report, where a surfing metaphor was used to describe the challenge to implement CIS: catching a wave. Our respondents in Hawaii Kaiser Permanente saw e-health as part of their future and were ready to embrace it. The instrument they were given was not state of the art. They persevered; it was a wild ride. What sustained them and the organisation was an extraordinary awareness and strength of belief in their culture, and its integration in a wider context of Hawaiian culture. At times that belief was tested and discrepant behaviour surfaced – nice, amiable doctors 'talked stink'. Dumped by the wave, they resolved to paddle out and try again, hopefully to do it differently and better.

CIS became the focus of a culture clash. It raised fundamental questions in participants' minds concerning the purpose and meaning of their work. Which mattered most: loyalty to the organisation or to the patients? How could these two be separated? This created a dilemma that would not go away. The poignant relief felt when CIS was officially withdrawn was not, we suggest, just from unloading a faulty product and the prospect of a better one. It also involved a recognition that certain key values had been saved and vindicated: the meaning of their work; why they elected to work for Kaiser; the organisation's culture; the commitment to prepaid group practice; to belief in 'caring for Hawaii's people like family'. CIS became, or at least came to be seen as, a threat to all of that.

Limitations of the study

Through the interviews we identified specific organisational processes associated with EMR implementation: the adoption decision, the unanticipated consequences, diversity, inter-regional differences, organisational culture, leadership, approaches to implementation, workflow analysis, healthcare teams, specialty differences, training and support, a magnification of errors, CIS team management, coping with change, time burden, previous IT applications, resistance and conflict. But, arguably, our most important finding lies not within such categories of aids and hindrances: it is in the weakness of that type of analysis. This weakness hinges on their essential ambiguity as aids *or* hindrances according to contextual factors, microscopic differences, different perspectives, and interests. Which is another way of saying that what facilitates or hinders implementation is contingent on an organisation's ecology. Ecology is not intended here as a dominant metaphor, but simply to capture the complex interdependence of forces at play. This all adds up to a questioning of approaches postulating 'organisational factors' as 'independent variables' affecting innovation. From a process perspective[72,73] there are no factors that in practice cannot be construed as facilitators and/or barriers, and none that could not, by sensitive leadership, or by interaction over time, be transformed from one to another. A strong culture may be a receptive or unreceptive context for a particular innovation. A weak and ailing culture may also be a receptive or unreceptive context. An innovation may be perceived as therapeutic or poisonous to a culture. The opposite causality is equally possible: a culture may promote or destroy innovation.

Validity of interview data

Critics of the adoption of second-generation CIS felt vindicated by its reversal. But the certainty of their convictions may have been exaggerated in retrospect. At the decision phase, all large-scale EMR systems were less developed and the decision to buy or build less clear; and the technical feasibility of scaling Epic was unresolved. A proper analysis of the adoption decision may not be feasible.

What might have been vaguely formed doubts at the decision phase may appear sound judgements in hindsight. It is part of the attribution effect to congratulate ourselves on being more right and sure than we really were. All of which signals caution concerning our ability to generalise findings and lessons from this type of research, or even to arrive at firm conclusions.

The implementation of CIS, or any other EMR, leads to a transient period of decreased production. This decline was very threatening to clinics already at maximum utilisation. Access in Hawaii was already at tipping point. 'At the time of selection we had to decide, "You know, it may go against us: what are we gonna do if they pick the other one (CIS): do we still wanna go first?" And the answer to that was "Yes".' If the answer had been 'No', how would CIS's career have been different? Would the same system have worked better if it had been implemented in a different region? Even if it had, would Hawaii have been any more successful when its turn for implementation came? Was Hawaii the right region to implement CIS? There is no simple answer. General rules derived from the intricate contingencies of one case might not apply to those of another. At least. after CIS, Hawaii was ready for EpicCare.

Success and failure revisited

We set out to answer three questions. How successful was the implementation of CIS in Hawaii? How did participants account for success or failure? And what were the organisational factors that helped or hindered the implementation? We are now in a position to address the third question one last time. But first we need to revise our terms of reference. What do we really mean by success? Success cannot be defined simply in terms of how many sites were using the application. On balance we think it unrealistic to classify CIS as either a success or a failure. It was a complex of micro-successes and micro-failures that do not add up to one grand conclusion. This complex whole can best be termed a learning process. We have argued that success also refers to the health of the organisation before, during and after the implementation. Many other dimensions of success could be added: financial, clinical, collective, personal.

Success or failure of EMR implementation is a long-term issue, which depends, ultimately, on the degree to which a health system succeeds in realising the theoretical advantages of the electronic record. But also, success and failure are socially negotiated judgements, not static categories.[1] They fail to capture the complexity of the partial CIS implementation in Hawaii. We need to revise our theoretical assumptions in this area. Evaluation of complex interventions like CIS is not a rational pre-, post-test procedure. What matters is how innovation mediates and is mediated; how it is managed, represented, handled, discussed. The before is not strictly comparable to the after, as the system changed through innovation. What phases did the implementation go through; what blocks and conduits were met and how negotiated? What new directions were taken? What did participants learn about themselves, their organisation, their assumptions; their culture? The success or failure of an EMR implementation will ultimately be determined by the participants' answers to those questions, what they learned from the experience, and how it affected their working relationships.

Appendix A: Facilitators and barriers to IT implementation and its effects on clinical care design

---

Introductions

Give business card to respondent

We are conducting an exploratory study of implementing the electronic medical record (EMR) in the Kaiser Permanente Hawaii.

The objective is to learn from leaders, change agents, clinicians and others about the facilitators and barriers to implementing EMR and its role in redesigning care processes.

We are also interested in any changes to chronic disease management that EMR has helped to introduce.

We are especially interested in differences in how organisational cultures mediate between planned and actual implementation of EMR (in the literature termed the 'implementation gap'); in any variation between sites in how they use EMR in practice; in the extent of integration of EMR and clinical practice; and in whether EMR has led to any significant changes in care management processes.

Through this pilot study we hope to get a clearer understanding of how physicians have responded to EMR implementation and associated efforts to redesign patient care.

This research may help us improve future EMR implementation.

Obtaining consent

May I have your permission to turn on the recorder before I ask for your consent to participate in the research?

Have you received a copy of your rights as a research participant, and an information and consent form? If you are satisfied with the information and wish to continue with the interview, please sign the form now, if you haven't already done so. Thank you.

Interviewee: .... Date: ....

Leaders, policy makers and researchers are concerned with what is termed the 'implementation gap'. That is, an observed discrepancy between planned and actual organisational change. We hypothesise that an organisation's culture mediates strongly between planned and actual change. If there are important differences between the cultures of organisations or units, we would expect to find corresponding differences in how a strategic planned change such as an EMR is implemented. Our interest in the implementation of the EMR, therefore, is to examine this hypothesis. I'd like to start by asking you about the culture of the organisation in which you work.

1 **Establish unit of analysis:** It would be helpful to establish first of all who we are talking about in this discussion – our unit of analysis if you like. Because I'd like you to pitch your answers at a level of generality that you feel comfortable with. Am I right in thinking that it would be mainly:
Prompt:
a   yourself and your immediate workgroup
b   the clinic as a whole
c   the Department
d   the Hospital
e   the Hawaii region.
Notes:

2 **Practice culture:** And how would you describe the culture of that unit/practice/department/hospital/region? What makes it unique in terms of the way things are done around here – what are regarded as normal behaviour and expectations; acceptable and unacceptable values and beliefs; even perhaps some of the underlying assumptions that inform what people think and do?
Prompt: Is it, for example:
a   like a family
b   entrepreneurial
c   bureaucratic
d   is efficiency of operation highly valued
e   other.
Notes:

3 **Cultural mediation:** Would you say that the culture of the unit/organisation(s)/region has affected how EMR was or is being implemented? In what ways?
Prompt:
a   pace of implementation
b   choice of initial implementation sites
c   presence of clinical leadership for EMR
Notes:

4 **Leadership:** A key factor relating to an organisation's culture is its leadership. Do you think that styles of leadership have influenced the implementation of EMR in this clinic/hospital/region?
   Prompt:
   a   senior staff provide highly visible leadership for EMR implementation
   b   leaders generate confidence that EMR will be implemented successfully
   c   effective leadership for EMR implementation has been lacking here
   d   clinicians have not needed leadership to implement EMR.
   Notes:

5 **Defining moments/critical events/turning points:** Have there been any defining moments in the implementation of the EMR: any critical event that marked a turning point in clinicians' interpretation and use of the system?
   Notes:

6 **Previous IT implementations:** (Draw a distinction between the technical characteristics of the EMR and its implementation.) How, if at all, has the experience of the EMR implementation been affected by previous IT implementations? e.g.:
   Prompt:
   a   expected that EMR would be better than previous systems
   b   confident that people would have learned not to replicate the same mistakes as occurred when implementing previous systems
   c   sceptical of the value of the new system
   d   dreaded the implementation.
   Notes:

7 **Use of EMR:** What changes has the implementation of EMR actually made to clinical practice or care processes? Has it changed:
   Prompt:
   a   how consultations are conducted
   b   how a clinician's work is organised
   c   how clinical work is coordinated between individuals/across sites
   d   automation of existing care processes
   e   redesign of care processes
   f   chronic disease management.
   Notes:

8 **Chronic disease management:** Would you say that the EMR is an effective vehicle to develop more effective chronic disease management programs (at unit/org/regional levels)? e.g. for:
   Prompt:
   a   diabetes
   b   asthma
   c   congestive heart failure
   d   depression
   e   other illnesses.
   Notes:

9 **EMR functionality:** Which, in your view, are the most useful aspects or functions of EMR to help to improve chronic disease management? e.g.:
Prompt:
a   electronic patient record
b   access to records from other clinicians and sites
c   tests and procedures ordering
d   diagnosis and treatment outcomes reporting
e   drug order entry
f   automated alerts and reminders
g   electronic communication with patients
h   health history.
Are there any other functions that would be helpful to improve chronic disease management, e.g. g or h above?
Notes:

10 **The new Epic system:** What are your thoughts about the decision to install a new Epic system to all Kaiser Permanente centres? e.g.:
Prompt:
a   in terms of integration
b   for chronic disease management
c   for individual healthcare
d   for population health.
Notes:

11 **Any other comments:** Can you think of anything else that might help us to learn from implementing the EMR in Hawaii?
Prompt:
a   Including anyone else that we should talk to.
Notes:

Thank you for taking the time to help us with our research. Please contact me if you think of anything else that you would like to add to our conversation. You have my card.

Reserve questions

12 **Facilitators to implementing EMR:** What in your view have been the main factors **facilitating** the implementation of the EMR in Hawaii? e.g.:
Prompt:
a   organisational culture supports quality improvement
b   previous electronic medical record or information system
c   supportive managerial and medical leadership.
Notes:

13 **Barriers to implementing EMR:** What in your view have been the main **barriers** to implementing the EMR in Hawaii? e.g.:
Prompt:
a   lack of financial and staff resources

   b   inadequacies of EMR
   c   doctors too busy to learn how to use it properly
   d   insufficient incentives
   e   too frequent change of electronic medical record or information systems
   f   doctors resist change
   g   other risks.
Notes:

14 **Positive or negative impact of EMR:** Would you say that EMR implementation has had only positive effects on clinical practice/care processes, or have there been any negative effects? e.g.:
Prompt:
   a   disruptions to practice management
   b   disruptions to patient care
   c   other.
Notes:

15 **Clinical integration:** Much is said about integration in healthcare systems in general, and in Kaiser Permanente in particular. What do you understand by the term 'integration'? What are the key integration priorities from your point of view?
Prompt:
   a   better or worse teamwork
   b   greater or less uniformity of care across providers
   c   closer or weaker liaison between primary and secondary care
   d   stronger or weaker regional identity
   e   stronger or weaker national Kaiser Permanente identity.
Notes:

Has EMR had any impact on integration, and in what ways?

16 **Acceptability of EMR:** What in your view are or were the key factors determining the acceptability of the EMR system in the unit/practice/department/hospital/region?
Prompt:
   a   clinicians were involved in designing the EMR
   b   a respected clinical champion was/is committed to EMR
   c   EMR is an important tool to improve clinical practice
   d   EMR is an important tool to improve chronic disease management in particular
   e   the EMR has the right functions to support care management processes
   f   staff will benefit from using the EMR.
Notes:

17 **Ability to implement EMR:** Would you say that practice members felt in a strong position to implement the EMR? Why?
Prompt:
   a   because clinical staff received adequate training

b   because adequate financial resources were committed to implementation and support
c   there was low resistance to change in the practice
d   people with the right technical knowledge were/are available to help with problems.
Notes:

18 **Alternatives to EMR:** To what extent are alternative systems to the EMR still in use (e.g. paper-based, or previous IT systems)?
Prompt:
a   not at all
b   occasionally
c   quite often
d   constantly.
Notes:

References

1   Aarts J, Doorewaard H, Berg M. Understanding Implementation: The Case of a Computerized Physician Order Entry System in a Large Dutch University Medical Center. *Journal of American Medical Informatics Association*. 2004; **11:** 207–16.

2   Anon. *Sidney Garfield Oral History: transcription of an interview*. The Permanente Archives; Undated.

3   Argyris C, Schon D. *Organizational Learning*. Reading, MA: Addison-Wesley; 1978.

4   Audit Commission. *For Your Information: a study of information management and systems in the acute hospital*. London: HMSO; 1995.

5   Bach P, Cramer L, Warren J, Begg C. Racial differences in the treatment of early-stage lung cancer. *New England Journal of Medicine*. 1999; **341:** 1198–1205.

6   Bachrach P, Baratz M. The Two Faces of Power. *American Political Science Review*. 1962; **56:** 947–52.

7   Bates DW. Using information technology to reduce rates of medication errors in hospitals. *BMJ*. 2000; **320**(7237): 788–91.

8   Bates DW, Leape L, Cullen D. Effect of computerized physician order entry and a team intervention on prevention of serious medication errors. *JAMA*. 1998; **280:** 1311–16.

9   Brennan T. Incidence of adverse events and negligence in hospitalized patients: results of the Harvard Medical Practice Study I. *New England Journal of Medicine*. 1991; **324:** 370–6.

10 Bryman A. *Quantity and Quality in Social Research*. London: Unwin Hyman; 1988.

11 Brynjolfsson E, Hitt L. Beyond computation: information technology, organizational transformation, and business performance. *Journal of Economic Perspectives*. 2000; **14**(4): 23–48.

12 Centers for Disease Control. *Diabetes Fact Sheet*. Altanta, GA: CDC; 1998.

13 Chall M. *Cecil C. Cutting, MD: History of the Kaiser Permanente Medical Care Program*. Berkeley, CA: Regional Oral History Office of the Bancroft Library; 1985.

14 Clark C, Fradkin J, Hiss R, Vinicar F, Warren-Boulton E. Promoting early diagnosis and treatment of type 2 diabetes. *JAMA*. 2000; **284:** 363–5.

15 Cutting C. *Annual Report, Kaiser Medical Care Program*; 1984.

16 Demarkis J, Beauchamp C, Cull W. Improving residents' compliance with standards of ambulatory care: results from the VA Cooperative Study on Computerized Reminders. *JAMA*. 2000; **284:** 1411–16.

17 Department of Health. *Building the Information Core: implementing the NHS Plan*. London: Department of Health; 2001.

18 Douglas M. *Purity and Danger: an analysis of concepts of pollution and taboo*. Penguin, Harmondsworth; 1966.

19 Epstein A, Ayanian J, Keogh J. Racial disparities in access to renal transplantation: clinically appropriate or due to underuse or overuse? *New England Journal of Medicine*. 2000; **343:** 1537–44, 2 p preceding 1537.

20 Evans R, Pestotnik S, Classen D. A computer-assisted management program for antibiotics and other antiinfective agents. *New England Journal of Medicine*. 1998; **338:** 232–8.

21 Fiscella K, Franks P, Gold M, Clancy C. Inequality in quality: addressing socioeconomic, racial, and ethnic disparities in health care. *JAMA*. 2000; **283:** 2579–84.

22 Foucault M. *Discipline and Punish*. London and Harmondsworth: Penguin; 1977.

23 Friedman C, Wyatt J. *Evaluation Methods in Medical Informatics*. New York: Springer-Verlag; 1997.

24 Gibbs W. Taking computers to task. *Sci Am*. 1997; **278**: 64–71.

25 Gregory JN. *American Exodus: the Dust Bowel Migration and Okie Culture in California*. New York and Oxford: Oxford University Press; 1989.

26 Halfpenny P. The Analysis of Qualitative Data. *Sociological Review*. 1979; **27**(4): 779–825.

27 Hammersley M. *What's Wrong with Ethnography? Methodological explorations*. London: Routledge; 1992.

28 Hendy J, Reeves BC, Fulop N, Hutchings A, Masseria C. Challenges to implementing the national programme of information technology (NPfIT): a qualitative study. *BMJ*. 2005; **331**: 331–6.

29 Hoyert D, Arias E, Smith BL , Murphy S, Kochanek K. Deaths: final data for 1999. In: *National Vital Statistics Report 49*. National Center For Health Statistics (US); 2001.

30 Humber M. National programme for information technology. *BMJ*. 2004; **328**: 1145–6.

31 Hunt DL, Haynes R, Hanna S, Smith K. Effects of computer-based clinical decision support systems on physician performance and patient outcomes: a systematic review. *JAMA*. 1998; **280**(15): 1339–46.

32 Huth O. *Raymond Kay, MD: History of the Kaiser-Permanente Medical Care Program*. Berkeley, CA: Regional Oral History Office at the Bancroft Library; 1985.

33 Institute of Medicine. *The Computer-based Patient Record: an essential technology for health care*. Washington, DC: National Academy Press; 1997.

34 Institute of Medicine. *Crossing the Quality Chasm: a new health system for the 21st century*. Washington, DC: National Academy Press; 2001.

35 Institute of Medicine. *Fostering Rapid Advances in Health Care: learning from system demonstrations*. Washington, DC: National Academy Press; 2002.

36 Institute of Medicine. *Priority Areas for National Action: transforming health care quality*. National Academy Press, Washington DC; 2003.

37 Ives ED. *The Tape-Recorded Interview: a manual for fieldworkers in folklore and oral history*. Knoxville, TE: The University of Tennessee Press; 1995.

38 Jessup M. Mechanical cardiac support devices – dreams and devilish details. *New England Journal of Medicine*. 2001; **345**: 1490–92.

39 Kaplan B. Development and acceptance of medical information systems: an historical overview. *J Health Hum Resour Adm*. 1988; **11**: 9–29.

40 Keene C. The Growing Demand for Information on Prepaid Group Practice. In: A.R. Somers (ed.) *The Kaiser Permanente Medical Care Program: one valid solution to the problem of health care delivery in the United States*. New York: The Commonwealth Fund; 1971.

41 Kohn L, Corrigan J, Donaldson M. *To Err Is Human: building a safer health system*. Washington, DC: National Academy Press; 1999.

42 Krippendorff K. *Content Analysis: an introduction to its methodology*. London: Sage; 1980.

43 Krishnamurti. *Krishnamurti Reader*. Harmondsworth: Penguin; 1954–64.

44 Latour B. *Science in Action: how to follow scientists and engineers through society*. Cambridge, Mass: Harvard University Press; 1987.

45 Legoretta A, Christian-Herman J, O'Conner R, Hasan M, Evans R, Leung K. Variation in managing asthma: experience at the medical group level in California. *American Journal of Managed Care*. 2000; **6**: 445–53.

46 Leonard K. Critical Success Factors Relating to Healthcare's Adoption of New Technology: A Guide to Increasing the Likelihood of Successful Implementation. *Electronic Healthcare*. 2004; **2**(4): 72–81.

47 Littlejohns P, Wyatt J, Garvica L. Evaluating computerised health information systems: hard lessons still to be learnt. *BMJ*. 2003; **326**: 860–63.

48 Lorenzi N, Riley R. *Organizational Aspects of Health Informatics: managing technological change*. New York: Springer-Verlag; 1995.

49 Lorenzi N, Riley R. Managing Change: An Overview. *Journal of American Medical Informatics Association*. 2000; **7**(2): 116–24.

50 Lukes S. *Power*. London and Basingstoke: Macmillan; 1974.

51 Marris P. *Loss and Change*. London: Routledge & Kegan Paul; 1986.

52 Marshall C, Rossman G. *Designing Qualitative Research*. London: Sage; 1989.

53 Miller R, Hillman J, Given R. Physician use of IT: results from the Deloitte Research Survey. *Journal of Health Information Management*. 2004; **18**(1): 72–80.

54 Miller R, Sim I. Physicians' use of electronic medical records: barriers and solutions. *Health Affairs*. 2004; **23**(2): 116–26.

55 National Audit Office. *The 1992 and 1998 IM&T strategies of the NHS Executive*. London: Stationery Office; 1999.

56 National Center for Health Statistics. *New Asthma Estimates: tracking prevalence, healthcare and mortality*. Hyattsville, MD: National Centre for Health Statistics; 2001.

57 National Heart Lung and Blood Institute. *Congestive Heart Failure Data Fact Sheet*. Washington, DC: National Institutes of Health; 1996.

58 National Institute of Mental Health. *Mental Disorders in America*. Washington, DC: HIHM; 2001.

59 NHS Information Authority. *NHS IA Strategic Plan for 2002–05*. Birmingham: Crown; 2002.

60 Partnership for solutions. *Better Lives for People with Chronic Conditions*. Baltimore, MD: Johns Hopkins University, Robert Wood Johnson Foundation; 2002.

61 Raymond B, Dold C. *Clinical Information Systems: achieving the vision*. Oakland, CA: Kaiser Permanente Institute for Health Policy; 2002.

62 Robinson TN. An evidence-based approach to interactive health communication: a challenge to medicine in the information age. Science Panel on Interactive Communication and Health. [Review]. *JAMA*. 1998; **280**(14): 1264–9.

63 Roethlisberger F, Dixon W. *Management and the Worker*. Cambridge, Mass: Harvard University Press; 1939.

64 Rogers E, Shoemaker F. *Communication of Innovations*. New York: The Free Press; 1971.

65 Rundall T, Shortell S, Wang M, Casalino L, Bodenheimer T, Gillies R *et al*. As good as it gets? Chronic care management in nine leading US physician organisations. *BMJ*. 2002; **325**: 958–61.

66 Schoen C, Doty MM, Collins SR, Holmgren AL. Insured But Not Protected: How Many Adults Are Underinsured? *Health Affairs*. 2005; **Web Exclusive, June 14, 2005**.

67 Schulman K, Berlin J, Harless W. The effect of race and sex on physicians' recommendations for cardiac catheterization. *New England Journal of Medicine*. 1999; **340**: 618–26.

68 Scott J, Mannion R, Davies H, Marshall M. *Health Care Performance and Organisational Culture*. Oxford: Radcliffe; 2003.

69 Scott JT, Rundall T, Vogt T, Hsu J. Learning from Kaiser Permanente's implementation of an electronic medical record in Hawaii: A qualitative study. *BMJ*. 2005; **331**: 1313–16.

70 Selznick P. *Leadership in Administration*. New York: Harper & Row; 1957.

71 Silverman D. *Doing Qualitative Research*. London, Thousand Oaks, CA, New Delhi: Sage; 2000.

72 Smillie JG. *Can Physicians Manage the Quality and Costs of Health Care? The story of the Permanente Medical Group*. New York: McGraw-Hill; 1991.

73 Smith Hughes S. *Clifford H. Keene: History of the Kaiser-Permanente Medical Care Program*. Berkeley, CA: The Regional Oral History Office of the Bancroft Library; 1986.

74 Smith Hughes S. *Lambreth Hancock: History of the Kaiser-Permanente Medical Care Program*. Berkeley, CA: The Regional Oral History Office of the Bancroft Library; 1986.

75 Songer T, Ettaro L. *Studies on the cost of diabetes*. Atlanta, GA: Centers for Disease Control; 1998.

76   Starr P. *The Social Transformation of American Medicine*. New York: Basic Books; 1982.

77   Stiell A, Forster A, Stiell I, Van Walraven C. Prevalence of information gaps in the emergency department and the effect on patient outcomes. *Canadian Medical Association Journal*. 2003; **169**(10): 1023.

78   Tang P, McDonald C. Computer-based patient-record systems. In: E Shortliffe, L Perreault (eds.) *Medical Informatics: Computer Applications in Health Care*. New York: Springer; 2001, p. 327–58.

79   Thompson D. *Transcript of an Interview with John G. Smillie*. Oakland, CA: The Permanente Archives; 1977.

80   United States Maritime Marine. Liberty Ship SS Robert E. Peary built in 4 days, 15 hours, 29 minutes. www.usmm.org/peary.html; (2000).

81   Wagner E, Austin B, Davis C, Hindmarsh M, Schaefer J, Bonomi A. Improving chronic illness care: translating evidence into action. *Health Affairs*. 2001; **20**(6): 64–7.

82   Weiss K, Sullivan S. The health economics of asthma and rhinitis: assessing the economic impact. *J Allergy Clin Immunol*. 2001; **107**: 3–8.

83   Whyte W. Interviewing in field research. In: R. Burgess (ed.) *Field Research: a sourcebook and field manual*. London: George Allen and Unwin, p. 111–22; 1982.

84   Young A, Klap R, Sherbourne C, Wells K. The quality of care for depressive and anxiety disorders in the United States. *Archives of General Psychiatry*. 2001; **58**: 55–61.

85   Schein E. Organizational Culture and Leadership. San Francisco: Josey Bass; 1985.

Index

access/identity, CIS 44–5
access to knowledge resources, EMR
    component 3–5
accountability
    CIS benefit 60–2
    Panopticon 62
administrative data, EMR component 3–5
adoption decision, CIS 120–1
applications/functions, EMR 3–5
approaches, implementation 89–92, 122
aptitude, CIS 103–4
automation, CIS 56–8

barriers, implementation 118–33, 142–7
benefits
    CIS 59–69
    EMR 3–5, 59–60
blame, CIS 73–5
budget, NPfIT 1

care delivery issues
    CIS 43–7, 125
    Pandora's Box effect 43–4, 70, 124
care management processes (CMP), US 6
care process innovation, CIS 54
CDSS *see* computer decision support
    systems
challenges
    EMR 2–3
    sociological 2–3
    technological 2–3
change management, CIS 95–6
choosing the right EMR 135
chronic disease management 5–6
    CIS 67–8
CIS *see* Clinical Information System
'Cisco Kid', CIS 65
clinic cultures, CIS 77–8
clinical care design, implementation
    effects 142–7
clinical decision support, EMR component
    3–5
Clinical Information System (CIS)
    access/identity 44–5
    accountability 60–2

accounting for successes/failures 71–
    117
adoption decision 120–1
aptitude 103–4
automation 56–8
benefits 59–69
blame 73–5
care delivery issues 43–7, 125
care process innovation 54
change management 95–6
chronic disease management 67–8
'Cisco Kid' 65
clinic cultures 77–8
Colorado/Hawaii 72–3
communication 63–4
conflict 112–16, 131–2
context 7
in context 58–9
culture issues 75–82, 96–8
decision making 62–3
decision to adopt 71–2
delay 36–7
development 36–43
e-conversion 54–5
e-literacy 98
efficiency, operational 106–9
EMR 59–60
experiences 35–70
experiences summary 69–70
failures 71–117, 119, 141
flexibility loss 47–9
Hawaii/Colorado 72–3
healthcare teams 99–101, 126
IBM 73–5, 115–16
identity/access 44–5
implementation 31–3, 35–70, 80–2, 89–
    92, 104–6, 122
implications, wider 133
In-Basket 49–51
incorporating 102–4
integration 56–8
interagency communication 63–4
Kaiser Permanente-IBM conflict 115–16,
    131–2
leadership 82–9, 128–30

learning experience 132–3
lessons learned 68–9
magnifying effect 43–7, 70, 124
MD telephone triage 55–6
medical staff-nursing staff conflict 116,
    131–2
operational efficiency 106–9
opportunity costs 105
organisational culture 75–82, 126–8
Panopticon 62
patient flow improvement 93–6
personal conflict 112–13, 131–2
pilot 92–3
product design issues 37–9
quality 64–5
readiness 96–9
regional-national conflict 113–15, 131–2
reported experience 69–70
resistance 111–12, 130–1
responses 65–6, 101–4
rigidity 47–9
scope of practice 45–7
site size issues 98–9
specialty differences 96–8, 123
specialty subcultures 78–80
successes 71–117, 119–20, 141
support 101–3, 123
team management 104–6, 124–5
teams, healthcare 99–101, 126
technical problems 121–2
telephone triage 55–6
templates 51–4
time burden 106–9, 125–6
training 101–3, 123
transformation 56–8
user responses 65–6, 101–4
visits 65–6
workflow analysis 93–6
clinical roles/responsibilities, managing
    136
CMP see care management processes
Colorado/Hawaii, CIS 72–3
communication, interagency, CIS benefit
    63–4
communication problems, NPfIT 41
communication support, EMR component
    3–5
components, EMR 3–5
computer decision support systems
    (CDSS), EMR component 3–5
conflict
    CIS 112–16, 131–2
    Kaiser Permanente-IBM 115–16, 131–2

managing 137
medical staff-nursing staff 116, 131–2
personal 112–13, 131–2
regional-national 113–15, 131–2
conversion, e-conversion 54–5
culturally informed responses,
    anticipating 137
culture issues
    catching a wave 139–40
    CIS 75–82, 96–8
    clinic cultures 77–8
    implementation 80–2
    organisational culture 75–82, 126–8
    specialty subcultures 78–80

decision making, CIS benefit 62–3
decision support, EMR component 3–5
decision to adopt CIS 71–2
design, clinical care, implementation
    effects 142–7
design problems, initial 135–6
disease statistics, US 5–6
document management, EMR component
    3–5

e-conversion, CIS 54–5
e-literacy, CIS 98
efficiency, operational, CIS 106–9
Electronic Medical Record (EMR)
    benefits 3–5, 59–60
    challenges 2–3
    choosing the right EMR 135
    components 3–5
    experiences 1–2
    implementation lessons 134–41
    key processes 135–40
electronic patient record, EMR component
    3–5
EMR see Electronic Medical Record
evidence, benefits 3–5
experiences, CIS 35–70

facilitators, implementation 118–33, 142–7
failures, CIS
    accounting for 71–117
    revisited 141
    summary 119
financial effects, NPfIT 41–2
flexibility loss, CIS 47–9
frustrations, managing 137
functions/applications, EMR 3–5

Hawaii/Colorado, CIS 72–3

Hawaii Kaiser Permanente, profile 6–7
healthcare teams
    CIS 99–101, 126
    implementation 99–101, 126

IBM
    CIS 73–5, 115–16
    Kaiser Permanente conflict 115–16, 131–2
identity/access, CIS 44–5
implementation
    approaches 89–92, 122
    barriers 118–33, 142–7
    CIS 31–3, 35–70, 80–2, 89–92, 104–6, 122
    clinical care design 142–7
    culture issues 80–2
    facilitators 118–33, 142–7
    healthcare teams 99–101, 126
    innovation diffusion 91
    key processes 135–40
    leadership 82–92, 128–30
    lessons for 134–41
    models 138–9
    NPfIT 41–2
    operational efficiency 106–9
    team management 104–6, 124–5
    teams, healthcare 99–101, 126
    time burden 106–9, 125–6
implications, wider, CIS 133
In-Basket, CIS 49–51
incorporating CIS 102–4
innovation, care process 54
innovation diffusion, implementation 91
innovation impact, previous IT 109–11, 131
Institute of Medicine (IOM), reports 2–3
integrated communication support, EMR component 3–5
integration, CIS 56–8
interagency communication, CIS benefit 63–4
international context 1–2
interviews, research 30–4
IOM see Institute of Medicine
IT-based medical care paradigm, reasons 2–3

Kaiser Permanente
    history 6–30
    Mojave Desert: 1933–1938; 8–10
    Grand Coulee: 1938–1941; 10–11
    World War II and the shipyards: 1942–1945; 11–14

Survival and reorganisation in the postwar era: 1946–1951; 14–17
Struggle for control 1952–1955; 17–21
Tahoe Agreement: 1955–1960; 21–3
Regional Management Teams 23–5
in Hawaii 25–8
1960s–present: a model for American healthcare? 28–30
Kaiser Permanente-IBM conflict, CIS 115–16, 131–2
key processes, EMR implementation 135–40
knowledge resources access, EMR component 3–5

leadership
    CIS 82–9, 128–30
    implementation 82–92, 128–30
    promoting responsive 137–8
learning experience, CIS 132–3
legacy systems, NPfIT 42
limitations of the study 140–1

magnifying effect
    care delivery issues 43–4, 70, 124
    CIS 43–7, 70, 124, 125
MD telephone triage, CIS 55–6
medical staff-nursing staff conflict, CIS 116, 131–2
models
    complex adaptive 139
    implementation 138–9

National Program for Information Technology (NPfIT)
    budget 1
    communication problems 41
    financial effects 41–2
    implementation 41–2
    legacy systems 42
    performance ratings 42
    timetable, implementation 42

operational efficiency, CIS 106–9
opportunity costs, CIS 105
organisational culture, CIS 75–82, 126–8

Pandora's Box effect, care delivery issues 43–4, 70, 124
Panopticon
    accountability 62
    CIS 62
patient flow improvement, CIS 93–6

performance measuring, EMR component 5
performance ratings, NPfIT 42
personal conflict, CIS 112–13, 131–2
pilot, CIS 92–3
practitioner order entry, EMR component 3–5
previous IT innovation impact 109–11, 131
productivity impact 136

qualitative research 30–2
quality, CIS benefit 64–5
quantitative research 31

readiness, CIS 96–9
reasons, IT-based medical care paradigm 2–3
references 148–51
regional-national conflict, CIS 113–15, 131–2
reliability, research 32–3
reported experience, CIS 69–70
reports, IOM 2–3
research
    interviews 30–4
    limitations of the study 140–1
    methodology 30–4
    qualitative 30–2
    quantitative 31
    reliability 32–3
    validity 32–3, 140–1
research context 2–3
resistance
    CIS 111–12, 130–1
    managing 137
resources access, EMR component 3–5
responses
    anticipating 137
    CIS 65–6, 101–4
rigidity, CIS 47–9

scope of practice, CIS 45–7
site size issues, CIS 98–9

sociological challenge 2–3
specialty differences, CIS 96–8, 123
specialty subcultures, CIS 78–80
statistics, US disease 5–6
successes, CIS
    accounting for 71–117
    revisited 141
    summary 119–20
support, CIS 101–3, 123

team management
    CIS 104–6, 124–5
    implementation 104–6, 124–5
teams, healthcare
    CIS 99–101, 126
    implementation 99–101, 126
technical problems, CIS 121–2
telephone triage, CIS 55–6
templates, CIS 51–4
time burden
    CIS 106–9, 125–6
    implementation 106–9, 125–6
timetable, implementation, NPfIT 42
training, CIS 101–3, 123
transformation, CIS 56–8
trends 2–3

UK, EMR experiences 1
US
    chronic disease management 5–6
    CMP 6
    disease statistics 5–6
    EMR experiences 1–2
user responses, CIS 65–6, 101–4

validity, research 32–3, 140–1
visits, CIS 65–6

WAVE 109–11
wave, catching a 139–40
wider implications, CIS 133
workflow analysis, CIS 93–6